CW01666165

THE INFINITY OF GRIEF

A handhold guide to support, heal and live while grieving

MARIE BROWN

THE INFINITY OF GRIEF - *A handhold guide to support, heal and live while grieving*

ISBN: 978 - 1 - 3999 - 9238 - 1

First published in Great Britain in 2024 through Amazon self-publishing service

This book contains general information about trauma and mental health based on the experience of the author. It is not meant as medical advice, diagnosis or treatment, and you must not rely on the information in this book as an alternative or substitute to medical advice from your doctor or other professional healthcare provider. If you have any concerns or questions regarding your health or that of your children or adults within your care, you should seek advice from your doctor. If you think you may be suffering from any medical condition, you should seek immediate attention from your doctor or other professional healthcare provider. You should never delay seeking medical advice, disregard medical advice or discontinue medical treatment based on information in this book. To the extent that you rely on any information in this book, you assume all risks involved in such reliance

Produced by samanthahoughton.co.uk

DEDICATION

Dale - the love of my life. I love you, always have, and always will.

Chloe, Chelsie, Jacob, Georgie, Arlo and Romeo. You are all my world; I love you all for infinity.

xxxx

TABLE OF CONTENTS

Authors Note ix

Praise For.... xi

Foreword xiii

I Am Me xvii

About The Author. xix

Words of Remembrance xxiii

Then and Now. xxvii

BEFORE: Your Loss. .1

Chapter 1: Time is Precious 3

Chapter 2: Loving All We Have 7

Chapter 3: Having the Gift of Time 9

Chapter 4: The Before, Dealing with a Diagnosis . . . 13

DURING: Grieving. 17

Chapter 5: No Choice? 19

Chapter 6: The Big Ask of Grief 23

Chapter 7: The Stages of Grief and Reaching For Help. . 29

Chapter 8: The Grief Club 35
Chapter 9: What Does Normal Mean? 41
Chapter 10: Intrusive Thoughts 45
Chapter 11: Triggers. 53
Chapter 12: Grief and Addiction. 59
Chapter 13: Love Hurts 65
Chapter 14: Suicide Grief 69
Chapter 15: Grief and Its Horrible Grief Friends . . . 83
Chapter 16: The Stillness of Grief 91
Chapter 17: Your Inner Strength 95
Chapter 18: Crying 99
Chapter 19: Driving Lessons of Grief 105
Chapter 20: Feelings Around Grief 109
Chapter 21: Respect Each Other's Grief. 117
Chapter 22: My Grieving Life 125
Chapter 23: Emotions 129

AFTER: When Some Time Has Passed 133
Chapter 24: Continuing Forward 135
Chapter 25: Live Your Life 137
Chapter 26: Positive Affirmations 139
Chapter 27: The Importance of Self-Care 141
Chapter 28: Do You 149

Chapter 29: Signs 153
Chapter 30: The Here and Now 157
Chapter 31: Getting to Know the New You. 161
Chapter 32: Coming Through the Other Side of Grief . 165

The After Me. 169
To My Family and Friends 171
Helplines and Support 173

AUTHORS NOTE

There is no right or wrong way to grieve. I wrote this book as a guide to help you understand grief.

No book should ever replace professional help that one may need.

I intend for this book to be a comfort, a handhold, a hug, and guidance in getting you back to feeling yourself again.

Love Marie x

PRAISE FOR...

"Wow, the emotions that came from me during the book; I can't praise you enough. It's absolutely brilliant, and I'm blown away. I wish every bereaved person had access to it right now."

Angela Michelback (funeral arranger)

"Your strength and determination to find ways to cope with painful and difficult times comes through in spades. I can feel how your love and positivity have and continue to support your precious family through the darkest times, keeping everyone afloat.

Your reflective words offer gentle suggestions for dealing with feelings and emotions, which is very powerful. I'm sure that reading about other people's experiences of grief will help them feel less alone, as it's clear that no one escapes grief.

You can dip into this book at any point and find words of comfort and wisdom. You have done a special and amazing thing."

Rachael Milczarek

FOREWORD

I am honoured to introduce Marie's book, which will help you understand how grief can impact people's lives and the emotions you may experience in grieving for your loved one, whatever the circumstances. I hope you can take some comfort from the words and experiences in the book and use this to help with your own infinity of grief.

Marie is a member of my family, and we have experienced many losses of our loved ones together over the years. Marie was always present after someone died; sometimes, being there is enough because of the importance of us all being together at such a sad time.

Marie is a calming person to be around. She is always thinking of others and has chosen, throughout her own grief, to help others by writing this book. I am sure it has also helped Marie. Marie has echoed the importance of self-care and taking time for me.

She told me, "Do what is right for you on that day," and I do.

Grief is like the ocean: It comes in waves, ebbing and flowing. Sometimes, the water is calm, and sometimes, it is overwhelming. There will be triggers for some, and we all experience it in our own way. It is such an individualised thing. Most importantly, there is support available, and you are not alone and never will be.

As a nurse for nearly twenty years, I have had a lot of experience in supporting patients and their families through dying; death and grief are a huge part of my daily life. I now work as a Community Specialist Nurse in Palliative Care.

People often ask me, "How do you do your job?"

There is no other job I would do. Not only do I make a difference to a person living with a life-limiting illness with their physical symptoms, but a big part of my role is supporting their emotional and social needs; it is a very holistic approach. I have the pleasure of getting to know them as people, and this often includes their families. It is a very patient-centred approach; they control the decisions that affect them and what we discuss. I help them make choices and support their fears by finding out what is important to them in life and when they die.

Understandably, I see a lot of sadness and anger from the people I meet, and often, what they don't realise is their grieving has already commenced. Their grieving may be for the person with the illness, their friends and family or a loss of independence, and not being able to carry out tasks that they used to do are all reasons life is changing beyond their control.

I have also had my own experiences of grief since I was a young teen. Each experience has been different for me, and yet I have found that no matter who the person is who has died, the overwhelming feelings of sadness and loss are the same. What I have found different is how overwhelming the feelings and thoughts can be depending on my relationship with them and how it impacts my family.

Seeing the difference I make in my role helps me with my own grief, and I feel very privileged to be able to do so. I work alongside people who are in their volunteering roles to share their own experiences of helping others, and this is what Marie is doing with her book.

Grief is the price we pay for love.xx

Warmest Wishes
Kelly Richardson

I AM ME

I want to be me.
Don't lose yourself.
I want to be the old me before grief.
But I am still me.
I want to do things the same way I did before grief.
But I am still me.
I want to be at peace like before grief.
But I am still me.
I want to be happy and hopeful.
But I am still me.
I can now work through the grief.
To still be me
I can still do the things I did before grief.
To still be me
I am hopeful and can see the light.
To still be me
I can heal and be at peace.
I am me.

ABOUT THE AUTHOR

My name is Marie, and I am fifty-six years old. I left school and trained to be a hairdresser. I had three children and continued hairdressing, and I have always loved working with people. I then felt I needed a change, so I went back to college to undertake counselling training. I left with newfound confidence to continue to help society. I went to a job rehabilitating people who had suffered brain injuries, allowing them to get back to a more productive and happy way of life after their brain injury.

It was then I found my dream job. I worked for over twenty years in hostels and supported housing with people who were homeless. I did assessments on why they had become homeless, helping them and their families if they had children, moving them into housing, and continuing to support them to prevent homelessness again. Although sometimes challenging due to the reasons they may have become homeless, including mental health, addiction, domestic violence and leaving prison, I met some amazing people throughout the years who taught me a lot through the way they coped when they were at their lowest, most vulnerable, and scared with no home. This was often through the most tragic crises or circumstances. They amazed me with their resilience and ability to carry on when feeling despairing when all seemed against them.

I remember a girl I once worked with who described her life as a jigsaw puzzle. Just as she tried to put the last piece in the puzzle, it was as if someone had scrambled all the pieces up. Hence, she felt like she would never be able to complete it, and her life would become chaotic again. It's easy to feel like this, but with support, a different thought pattern, and realising we are in control, we can all put in the final piece to have the self-love and the kindness we all deserve - living a life we are happy in. It can take time, but we can all achieve it.

I was going to write a book years ago when I lost my mum, but it didn't happen as the timing wasn't right. My counselling training was after losing my mum, which I believe gave me a lot of coping strategies to help me through my grief.

So why am I writing it now? I am in the depths of grief again and realise I must navigate my way through at the same time as surviving life, just like the hundreds of people's tragic stories I have heard over the years. We all desire to share our feelings, to get through it together, and to achieve a life we feel happy with that feels worth every breath.

I still remember so vividly my experience of grief when I lost my own mum. I recall those feelings and how they changed and affected me. Also, how I came out on the other side, continuing to live a life I enjoyed when, at the time, I did not think would ever be possible again. I remember leaving the hospice and feeling surreal like I was two steps back from everyone and everything going on. I was thirty-two years old with three young children and needed my mum. How would I survive? The waves of grief taught me that I had to keep dealing with it, which was another shock. The anger that, yes, the world around us carries on, with a piece of ourselves missing, which we must rebuild as we fight to find ourselves again.

I have since lost many family members and friends over the years, finding myself in many situations before, during, and after they pass away, all trying to get out of the tangled web of grieving and carry on with life.

I hope this book helps you through this and helps you learn that you can live a happy, fulfilled life and laugh and enjoy yourself without guilt or any other emotion. We do not need to hang on to move forward, even though we are carrying our grief around with us like unwanted baggage.

I feel I have a life worth living and want to live it to the fullest, as I deserve it. With all the grief journeys I have been on, I can share with you some of the ways I have dealt with this, enabling me to always move forward, maintain a positive outlook, and still feel well and happy.

WORDS OF REMEMBRANCE

When my mum passed away twenty-four years ago, there was no social media. Local newspapers had a special page for announcing births, deaths and marriages. I always thought it odd to have these next to each other in the paper. You would call the newspaper and tell them what you wanted them to print regarding your loved one passing away. Anyone could do this and leave words of remembrance, but only after the initial details of the funeral place, date and time were given by the funeral home doing the arrangements. This was how loved ones told the world about one of these big life events. It seems odd now that we use social media and let everyone know as much or as little as we want to.

As I was writing my book, my friend, who was also a close friend of my Mum, gave me an envelope she had found after Mum had passed away. In it, she had saved all the newspaper cuttings about Mum - the words my sister, brother, and I had published. There were also all the other words of condolence friends and family had put in the paper to show their love.

When I reread these words that I hadn't read for years and years, it made me realise how every word on that paper was still as true then as it is now; I felt every word as if time had stood still, transporting me back, the grief still locked away inside me, becoming part of me, changing me and going through and coming out the other side - the power of words.

Grief changes us; it is painful and becomes part of us, but it doesn't have to take us. We have the ability to find within ourselves the strength to continue, as if the loss of our loved one's strength embeds in us to make them proud and get us on the right side of it, to continue our own lives to our fullest potential.

ROBINSON, Helen, a dear mum.
It broke our hearts to lose you,
But you did not go alone,
A part of us went with you,
The day God called you home.
A million words won't bring you back,
We know because we've tried,
Neither will a million tears,
We know because we've cried.
No one sees the broken heart,
That lies behind the smile,
No one knows the loneliness,
That's with us all the while,
Silent tears do gently fall,
That others do not see,
For a kind and loving mother,
Who meant the world to us.
We watched you suffer,
We watched you sigh,
All we could do was just sit by,
When the time came we suffered too,
You never deserved what you went through.
If you have a mother,
Love her while you may,
Because we wish with all our hearts,
We had our mum today.
Nothing in this world could ever replace,
Our loving mum with her smiling face,
Someone to turn to kind and true,
One in a million that was you,
The best mum in the world. Nanight mum.
All our love forever. — Marie, Steven, Karen, and Dale. xxxxx

THEN AND NOW

My first experience of losing someone was at the age of fourteen. It was 1981, and I came home from school to a house full of aunties and cousins, and my Mum was crying. She told me that my grandad had passed away. The first thing I remember is walking into an atmosphere I had not felt before. There was heaviness, stillness, silent tears, and a harrowed look on their faces. I had not seen this before: the look of grief. It was a combination I now know to be one of shock, sadness and an inability to process it all.

A relative told me to go upstairs, which I felt relieved about. I did not know how to be or react as it was new to me. Back then, people dealt with it with an almost "out of sight, out of mind" approach. After that moment, a family member shared a couple of practical facts with me regarding why my Mum and Dad would not be at home the day of the funeral when I got back from school.

I wasn't allowed to attend the funeral; I can't remember if I asked to go, but I knew it wasn't an option. A minister friend of mine said that he believes age is not a barrier when it comes to attending a funeral. He said it is the final goodbye, a time to be together with family and friends, to allow ourselves to move on to the next stage of grieving.

It's a personal decision to make. After we lost my son-in-law more recently, we decided that the children wouldn't attend as they were very young. Still, knowing they would need to say goodbye to move forward, we held a private family gathering. We walked to a spot where he had played as a child, and the children all let off helium balloons and said goodbye. They felt the closeness of being supported and held as they said goodbye. We explained that he was now a star in the sky. It was very moving, and the children understood what was happening. It was their special time to say goodbye, leaving them free to move into their next phase of grief.

Whatever way you do things, if anyone isn't attending the funeral, I think it's important to do something to mark saying goodbye to then allow us to keep moving forward. It's amazing how far this has come, with funerals being streamed live through links to other family members and friends who may be anywhere in the world. Or if, for any reason, someone cannot attend the funeral.

I wasn't asked how I was or how I felt as a teenager, and I didn't ask how anyone was feeling either after that day. My grandad was just gone and I missed him so much. For the first time, my family was different. Knowing I was loved by my family, being a teenager who always wanted to be with my mates, and being in my school routine, brought me through it.

It was different back then; no one spoke of feelings or emotions or asked if anyone was struggling. There appeared to be a get-on-with-it attitude; others considered it a weakness when speaking out. Men did not cry. Thankfully, this has changed, and we are ourselves and bringing our children up to understand the benefit of being open with how we feel.

I knew my family would never have hurt me intentionally. My mother had lost her father and would have been heavily grieving, but from that day, I would have never known anything was any different. I never heard my Mum and nana speak of how they felt or their sadness at what I know was a devastating loss to them. They kept their grieving hidden from us, as a way of protecting us. They left us to deal with everything alone as we tried to figure out how we were feeling, and most of the time, we buried it because we didn't know how to process it.

It is hugely different now, and we are encouraged to speak up about our feelings. This makes us feel less lonely about our grief. Although we still do some grieving in private, this is needed to process our emotions. Times have evolved, so it's okay for us to speak up. All this is a positive for us grievers, as we talk and share how circumstances make us feel, not feel alone, realise the importance of saying goodbye, and make a funeral more personal. We approach death differently now; we can celebrate the person's life. Speaking openly allows us to grieve to come out the other side of it and let go of the pain.

BEFORE

YOUR LOSS

CHAPTER ONE

TIME IS PRECIOUS

I have learnt over the years that if we have precious time with a loved one, knowing they are not going to be with us before long can make an enormous difference to our grieving process. This time is like gold; it need not be months or weeks. It could be only hours. I know it's hard to think straight in these situations with the stress of losing someone you care about at the forefront of your mind. However long the time is, use it wisely, and make the time to see this person as much as possible.

It's surprising what you can fit into an already busy routine when needed; you can use this time to resolve any unsaid issues and be at peace with yourself and them if required. Use this time to tell your loved one how much you care about them and how you will still achieve things you want to make them proud. It really helps to say this to the person while they are still here. If you find it difficult to say these things or voice anything unresolved, write them a note or a letter they can read, or someone else can read them. If the person is still here but really poorly or heavily sedated on medication, they will still hear your words, so you know they have heard what you want to say. Even if people are too poorly to respond they can still hear you.

When the time comes and your loved one passes, having no regrets about doing what you can in the last stages is one less thing to deal with when the grieving process begins. I remember when I lost my mum, I reflected after some time and thought if we hadn't cared for her and done all we had done for her at that extremely difficult time when she was here, to live with that alongside the devastating loss we all felt, would have weighed really heavy - so if you have the chance, always do what you feel you need to before it's too late.

Of course, we can all only do what we can, depending on our circumstances and what that allows, so we should never feel guilt for what another has done or can do. This can, of course, come with other difficulties, especially if, for example, we have young children or are working and just doing the normal things we have to fit into our busy lives. Give yourself space to think about the prognosis and realise that, like everything, the situation will change. Don't let the time slip away wishing you had done or said things you wish you had.

Trying to get the balance right can also be difficult. Be gentle with yourself; we can all only do what we can, and it's important to realise this. We are of no use to ourselves or others if we are not looking after our wellbeing. We don't need to take on guilt for looking after ourselves. I think, in general, it is becoming more recognised that this is a key factor in being able to help others; it can be something as simple as not giving up a weekly coffee date with a friend. We can always adapt these situations to fit into the busy time of looking after a loved one. An in-person meeting could change temporarily to a phone call, if necessary. Still, this time of chatting with your friend and being able to offload or have conversations about different things can be invaluable.

I think the normal things that we often take for granted can make you realise that they are actually the things that are really important. So it's not anything special you need to do with the person you love; it is just being present and together, and that's enough.

CHAPTER TWO

LOVING ALL WE HAVE

In my grieving process, I've often thought of times in the past when I thought I didn't realise how special my life was and that I may have possibly taken things for granted, including the special people in my life. I just thought it would be like that forever, and they would always be around.

I had lots of people in my life, and I have now lost them. After dealing with grieving lots of times, I have realised that we are here now, with our loved ones and friends around us. This is our now life.

I have read that people who took their own lives do so as they feel it's the only way to get out of how they are feeling. They didn't want to die but felt there was no alternative to their thoughts and pain and hopelessness. In these circumstances, we have to remove the unanswered questions and guilt from ourselves to allow ourselves to heal and find peace after pain.

My daughter said to me a year after her husband had passed away that she wanted to find more peace that year, and I felt that too, and we continue to work towards it.

None of us know what tomorrow will bring, so to process grief when we lose someone is paramount; I am giving myself permission to live and be thankful for all I have now. As I try to be the best I can, it can be difficult as grief turns up unexpectedly in our minds, but as time passes and the moments in between the grieving get a little longer, make these thoughts kind to yourself.

I remember someone once telling me to sit, close my eyes, and think of all I have in my life - my family, friends, people I love, my home, and everything positive. Now, for a second, please open your eyes and imagine it all gone; you will feel different about all you have at this moment in time.

The moral is to never lose sight of what we have now, be grateful for this moment, and cherish what we have and our relationships. Knowing everything becomes a memory will help us not crave what isn't important and to hold on to what is.

CHAPTER THREE

HAVING THE GIFT OF TIME

Whether we know a death will happen or not, the shock can affect the grieving process. A mind cannot take in all the thoughts that come with losing a person and what grieving may or may not bring while a person is still here. That's why grieving takes time, and new thought patterns and habits must be worked through to cope with this new life that's been thrown at us after our loved one has passed away.

It is important to focus on what is happening now and be present. Although we try to prepare ourselves for the loss if the situation allows it, it is important not to let this overtake the quality time we have left with the person.

The physical side of anticipating loss, body aches, and tension felt in the head and throughout your whole body is all normal and is something I never knew existed. Self-care is important during this to help you cope with the ever-changing times.

When I lost my mum and, for a long time after, I would pick up the phone as if to ring her and then remember that she wasn't there as we had spoken every day previously. Losing someone broke our daily routines and habits, which was something I hadn't even thought of being part of my grieving; it left us trying to fill the void with something else. Keep up these routines and cherish them.

We will have many thoughts in trying to prepare for the loss, some of which won't even happen, so I stress the importance of focusing on the present to keep making special memories and enjoying the time left you have together. Delay things that seem important but can wait. If you have this time, use it wisely. Those beautiful memories when a loved one is not here are all we must grip hold of when they are gone.

My mum loved Elvis, so when she was terminally ill in bed upstairs, we arranged a garden party at her home for all close family and friends to attend. It took some planning and gave us a positive focus. We had the most wonderful afternoon all together, listening to him sing her favourite songs. We took lots of photos to have treasured pictures of a special time. Again, it brought strength and comfort from being around people who care and seeing her smile brings me happiness now.

It doesn't matter how big or small creating these memories is; it is a blessing to be able to do so, knowing that things will change, but the memories will last a lifetime. Make time to reminisce, talk of things you enjoyed together, revisit spent magical moments, and listen to your favourite music together. Tell each other how you feel.

CHAPTER FOUR

THE BEFORE, DEALING WITH A DIAGNOSIS

While writing my book, my Dad and his fiancé rang to see if I was in so they could visit. There was nothing unusual about their request until they came to my house, and everything changed. It's mad how you know something bad has happened or is happening before someone speaks a single word or there is a look you don't want to see. You know, when the words come, it will be bad news, and things will change, and on this occasion, it resulted in me crying before they even spoke.

"Please don't tell me something bad," I said as if I could stop time and save myself from pain.

They looked at each other, and it was as if time stood still until I told them to tell me, and they said that my Dad had cancer. The shock, sadness, and the unknown future of what this meant spiralled into a deep sadness. They were calm, supportive and seemingly strong as they had had time to process this information and create a story of hope. Being strong in reality is massive as it takes a lot from you while fearing the unknown and how things will be.

It is important not to let your thoughts overtake you at this time. Being present is a gift. Be mindful of any information you receive at the time, digest it, and prepare for the next day of the road ahead. It is amazing, as humans, what we can deal with if we follow this process and do not try to control what is out of our control. There will be lots to cope with as the thoughts of others we have lost and what will become flood into our minds, such as not wanting my Dad to suffer, seeing and feeling the pain of others around us, and being fearful of the next step that we'd face. Taking it one day at a time allows us not to second guess what may happen.

My Dad, who's never not been in my life, was thrown into a whirlwind of my thoughts about him and my childhood mixed with fear and sadness knowing how ill he was. How ironic that I'm writing a book on grieving with my Dad still alive but having the fear of death and having to grieve him slapping me in the face again. I realise I have felt these feelings before. Our minds try to process what's going on, ultimately digging deep, and I realise he is still alive. He is so much bigger than a diagnosis. If you looked at my Dad, you wouldn't know he was ill; I could see in his eyes his pain in having to tell me.

It's hard not to let grief consume you and to keep your thoughts above water, thoughts that want to drag you down to an unmanageable level. However, a day-by-day approach helps this, as it's a new day every day and a chance to brush yourself down and start your thought process for that day. Of course, this isn't easy, but we must continue like this to be able to cope, to be supportive, and to run our lives alongside the devastating news.

Life is again put into perspective, demonstrating how delicate and precious it is and how we should breathe and remember this.

It made me realise, as I'm still grieving my son-in-law, that lots of the before someone passes and after emotions during grieving can feel the same. The knot in the stomach as you will it to untangle, the sadness, the anger, the fear of the unknown, the vulnerability and the difficult conversations we must work through. We constantly give ourselves advice to help us move forward to cope with what emotion comes up. We can do this as long as we breathe; we have the ability. We are not just our thoughts; we can change them and give ourselves the love we deserve. Knowing we want to be supportive; we can gain strength in the before process. We need to be the best we can be.

It is important around this time to have supportive people around you; we are extremely lucky that my Dad's fiancé is calm and caring and relays all information to us as it happens and keeps us in the loop; this is invaluable to help deal with the process. Naturally, fear of the unknown eats away at us as it tries to dominate our thoughts and sends us spiralling with limited knowledge and information.

Communication is key to helping this, so if someone else is going to the medical appointments and finding out the information firsthand, find ways that work for you so you know what's happening. Also, remember that the medical team dealing with this is the expert, so ask questions; they will constantly keep putting things in place to help you through the different scenarios you will face. You aren't alone in dealing with it all.

This is happening in my life right now, but we must stay focused and positive. I›m trying not to entertain any other emotion at the moment if it dances its way into and out of my thought process. Day by day is the way forward.

Palliative care describes the physical, psychological, and social care and support given to someone with a terminal illness. Many services are available to help you through this. Your GP, nursing team and health and social care team members are there to guide you, support you and hold your hand through this hard and stressful process. They work closely with all services in your community for the best possible care for your loved one.

DURING

GRIEVING

CHAPTER FIVE

NO CHOICE?

There is no stopping grief. When you lose someone you love, you are thrown into the grieving process right there and then at that moment. We have no choice, a process forced upon us like no other, stirring up emotions in us, some we never knew existed or felt before, making us feel vulnerable. It feels like all our emotions, old and new, are thrown into a washing machine, not knowing which one will come out of our brains first. We try to put them in an orderly queue and work through them along with a million thoughts as we attempt to come to terms with the loss. It leaves us feeling exhausted physically and mentally.

We must never underestimate the power of grief and how it takes its toll on us. We must recognise early in the process the need to be kind to ourselves to stop us from going under in this new world we find ourselves in, especially during the early days of grieving. When we allow ourselves the time to know our new grieving self and work through our thoughts to feel steady again, we can face what we need to continue our own life with grief walking alongside us to feel peace again. We can guide ourselves to where we feel we have a choice again, remembering we can control our thoughts and feelings. Grief will not always feel so consuming.

It's helpful to stop fighting against it and to work with whatever grief throws at us: the new feelings, the new choices, the new decisions, and our new life.

Angela's Story

My name is Angela; I have been in the funeral business for the last twenty-four years. My first real insight into the funeral service was when Marie's Mum, Helen, lost her long, hard battle with cancer. I remember that moment when I realised I had a deeper interest in the business, which I now know is my passion.

For me, the role of a funeral arranger is somebody who is warm, kind, caring and full of information and knowledge, mainly all the options that are available to make this very special day go ahead in a way that is not only very important to tribute the life of your loved one but also important for you and your journey after the day of the funeral. When having to arrange a funeral, many people have absolutely no idea where to start.

And that's where my role begins. It is an honour and a privilege when others entrust me with the care of somebody's loved one.

And carry on that care, helping and guiding the bereaved through what could be the most difficult time in their lives. From the first contact with a bereaved person, it is my responsibility to ensure them that we are here to help and guide them through all the necessary planning and organising while keeping them fully informed every step of the way.

My advice is: if you think it, then say it: your loved one's funeral service is only as good as the information you give. Fond memories, anecdotes, and wonderful stories are the essence of what keeps somebody alive. Never feel rushed and pressured to make a quick final decision.

CHAPTER SIX

THE BIG ASK OF GRIEF

Grief holds no plan, no diary, and no time to make a date with your emotions. It will keep turning up unannounced, and we are expected to deal with it forever. What a big ask of us, grief. We step up constantly, dealing with what it asks of us, navigating emotions we haven't felt physically and mentally before - like a game of brain Olympics. Our thoughts juggle our old life with our new grief life at the side, trying for them to meet on the same path. It asks us to constantly work through our feelings without considering our wellbeing or if we are exhausted. Grief is selfish, turning up and ruining the plans we have. It judges us if we have a good day, making us feel guilty.

Feeling the anger, a rage we have never felt surprises us as we don't even recognise our personalities and self-worth. Some days, it zaps us of all our energy - leaving us sitting numb, emotionless, and paralysed by the strain of grief. Grief makes us feel desperate; we hate our new grief life, and we feel we can't do it.

We long to run smoothly again and feel our steps are lighter and not wading through mud. In the early days, we had to do this daily, hour by hour, minute by minute. How amazing are we?

Sometimes, we must remember that it can be exhausting to do alone and know when to reach out. It's always okay to do this. I find a lot of the time people don't realise they stop asking if we are okay, checking in on each other as we are all scurrying around trying to be okay. We need to know if we are not dealing with stuff as we feel we should and remember the importance of communicating with others how we are.

We may just need to pick up our phone and chat with a friend or take ourselves out for a walk. A night out can distract from grief, but sometimes, we may need more. It is always okay to ask for help, so go to the GP or join support groups. You sometimes just have to push through the grief. Find what works for you moving forward. Remember, there is no right or wrong way, but if there is a feeling of not coping and struggling daily, reach out.

Always remember we are bigger than grief. As much as grief throws at us, we are there living it, feeling it, changing it, doing it, jumping through one emotion and then another. No thought pattern stays the same. We feel ourselves build back up and leave the harshness and pain grief brings behind as we continue to walk forward.

Gary's Story

The meaning of grief is intense sorrow, especially caused by someone's death.

Having lost my mother and wife, Teresa, all within the last nine months has sent my mind somewhere where it's never really been. I appreciate that death affects us all in different ways, and I have realised that maybe being the eldest sibling, being a husband, a father, and a brother can make things more difficult. As well as all the thoughts and emotions going through my head and trying to make sense of it all is one thing, but I also feel a responsibility and a need to stay strong for others and the need to make sure they are okay. A younger sister, my niece, who was very close to my Mum, and my siblings, have also lost two people very close to them in quick succession. I wonder whether having this responsibility to ensure others are okay is a positive or negative. Does it help me, or does it make my situation more difficult? My opinion is it's both. I feel helping others also helps me get through this difficult time, but it also upsets me more like an extended grief. So, how has grief affected me regarding my wife? Apart from the obvious, which is the sadness of a loss, the tears, etc., suddenly there is a physical void and empty space where the person is no longer there to touch, to talk to or to hold; you wake up in the morning, and there is no one to say good morning too or make a cup of tea for. You come home from work, again with no one there to ask you how your day has been or to have a meal with. You go to bed with no one to say, "I love you", no kiss goodnight, and it was not until my wife had gone that I realised how much these sorts of things meant or how much I miss not just her but these things we shared.

All these thoughts go through my head daily, and still, after six months, I miss her as much as I did the first day, night, and week. It's like a constant drain on your body, almost like you have lost a limb. Then there is guilt. Did I tell her how much I loved her enough? Did I do all I could for her? Am I doing all I can now for the family? I could have told her more or done more for her. The guilt is always there, which, rightly or wrongly, sometimes makes me feel guilty, and I torture myself, wishing I had done or said more. Some of the things I do daily are to ask myself what Teresa's or my Mum's opinion would have been and what they would have thought. I don't know if I will ever feel less sad and guilty. People will tell you time is a great healer, and maybe one day I will come to terms with my wife's and mother's death, but I am not sure the feelings will ever go away. As such, I might just come to terms with my thoughts.

Grief has also affected my view on death. I was always afraid of dying, and I don't know why, but I don't feel afraid anymore, and as strange as it sounds, I will be happy to join my wife again one day.

Finally, it surprised me how grief has affected my emotions. There is no set pattern, but I think about my Mum and wife every day. Sometimes, they are happy thoughts, sometimes sad, and I cry, which can be in private or in conversation; I find talking about it makes me feel very emotional and nearly always brings a tear and a lump to my throat. Then, for all that have lost someone, you have times which can be very difficult, like the first Christmas without them, birthdays, holidays, Valentine's Day, or the anniversary of their death; these all bring back memories which contain happiness, grief, guilt, and sadness.

It is the most difficult situation I have ever found myself in, and I am sixty-two years of age. Having to cope with grief is not nice. Still, we have no option but to deal with it because that's what my Mum and wife would have wanted, and that helps me cope and carry on knowing that although they are not here, I am doing something they would have wanted and of course, the love that will always be there.

CHAPTER SEVEN

THE STAGES OF GRIEF AND REACHING FOR HELP

Just after I had lost my Mum, I did a year's foundation course in counselling at Loughborough College. I didn't realise at the time how beneficial this was to my own grieving. In effect, my studying taught me not only how to help others going through trauma but also how to use the new things I was learning to help myself. Using the processes on myself, I think, saved me and helped me work through my grief to be able to continue and then find a way of living joyfully. I have since learnt this is called post-traumatic growth.

I realised after losing all the people in my life that the same core things for coping were very similar. Even though we are all different, it was a process we had no choice but to go through. It had to be worked through to try living our lives as well, knowing grief will always be by our side like a friend we don't want. But we must find a way of dealing with and doing life again while this unwanted friend chips and chats away at our thoughts and emotions, and working through it like unwanted homework forces us to be experts in dealing with emotions. We need to find ways of coping by trying to unscramble it in our unique brains to deal with it when we can't ever imagine laughing or enjoying ourselves again.

One part of the study was to write a weekly journal. I now realise that getting these feelings out of my head onto paper was extremely helpful. We did some grief training, and this is where I came across the gestalt cycle of grief; this was the first I had learned of the stages of grief we all go through:

Denial
Anger
Bargaining
Depression
Acceptance

I believe that there are lots and lots of other branches that come off these stages, forming a big grieving tree, such as the feeling of loneliness, of needing to pick up the phone to speak to them, wanting to hear their voice and lots of things personal to us that make up part of our grieving. It's normal to keep slipping in and out of different stages on the wild ride grieving takes us on as we constantly deal with it. I think we are all familiar with the main stages of grief headings, but sometimes it feels like a million and one little things we must keep dealing with, leaving us feeling overwhelmed and it all hard to manage.

We must all work through the stages and get to know ourselves on a whole new level. We must be aware that we must feel each stage; it's almost impossible to rush. It feels like we want to be over all the hard, draining feelings, but I know from experience that not working through them means they keep reoccurring, making it harder. Dealing with how it makes us feel is sometimes enough; some feelings we haven't felt before will feel alien to our whole body. We often question if we need help if we can't complete the process alone. We are all unique, and some can't, some can; it's not a competition; one is not right, and one is not wrong.

I had some telephone counselling sessions that I didn't find that helpful, but for others, it was extremely beneficial. I think the point I'm trying to make is that grieving is hard, and what works for one may not work for another, and that's okay.

One of the reasons to help you decide if you may need to look into receiving external help like counselling or a support group (I did find a support group that was hugely beneficial for me), is if you feel stuck on part of your grieving cycle. As I said, it's perfectly normal to slip in and out of these stages, but to be stuck on one part of it, for example, anger and not be able to work through it or move out of that stage or the stages are constantly flipping back and forth for you to work through, or you are feeling abnormal thoughts that you can't deal with, or you feel suicidal or just not coping reach out.

You are not alone. It's not a failure to ask; it's just part of your healing process to get to a place of peace and come out the other side. If this means someone helping you along to do this, you should be so proud of yourself for recognising this and doing something about it. Nothing in the grieving process stays the same as you will be aware of, let this be known to yourself that on the other side of it there is hope and peace. During dark days when you cannot see the light, keep moving forward even if you must do this day by day, hour by hour. If you can't work through it yourself, speak up; it will free you from dealing with it alone, give you a sense of relief, and allow you to move forward.

Also, this shows the importance of checking in on each other if someone we know finds it difficult to ask for help to reassure each other along our journeys. To realise we are in it together, but our individualism is what makes it different for each of us, as our relationship with the person we have lost is unique. When we are struggling, they may be feeling different things or be at different stages in grieving to be empathetic towards each other.

It's important to respect this and try and talk openly about it, or there is a risk it can cause conflict, and the grief can rip through, tearing families and friendships apart. It shows how important communicating is and not presume we know someone's feelings to empathise with each other to come together to help each other heal.

When I lost my son-in-law, who took his own life, one of the important parts of our ongoing healing was simply just checking in on each other and respecting how each other was feeling. Talking as a family, we are all still as close as we ever were, including us all with his family. We have carried each other along in the dark, desperate times of grief just simply by doing this; the comfort of knowing you have a family's support is everything, so always check in on each other and be available to help carry someone along if they need it.

If you feel alone or don't have the support of family or friends and are struggling, reach out. Your GP can help you find support groups or help you work out a way forward that suits you. I know it's hard, but speaking out is key to moving forward. Knowing it will benefit you, let it give you the confidence to do this. For you not to feel alone, sometimes it may not be professional help we need, picking up the phone and arranging to see someone we haven't seen for a while may be enough, whatever the reason, always reach out. There are hands to lead us. Still, we sometimes must make the first move.

THE STAGES OF GRIEF I AM WORKING THROUGH AND THE EMOTIONS I HAVE FELT

CHAPTER EIGHT

THE GRIEF CLUB

We are all now part of the same grief club, a place you only belong to if you have dealt with a loss and where you can empathise with anyone else in it, knowing how hard it is. The grief club is a club people are trying to get out of not in and where you must work to feel free from it.

I want this book to feel as though it's the same as having your friend to talk to, so you know you are not alone in this horrible world of grieving. We have no choice to be in a club that we didn't want to be part of. The club no one wants to be in, and you're only able to get a membership by losing someone you cared about. The criterion is grief - as you try to figure out ways to escape and be how you were before.

Truthfully, we are never the same again, and we now must survive this painful journey to get to the goal of feeling comfortable in the club. I want to make you feel as though you aren't going crazy to help you through the grieving process, working through the changes our minds go through, and being able to ride the emotional tsunami wave that happens when a loved one passes away. We can do this together; we can make our grief club one that we can come away from, and although we must keep re-visiting it, we can go there when we want to and not feel like we can't get away from it.

We should use our friends and family, who are now also members of this club, to communicate openly and support each other. When one manages to step out of it for a bit, they should share what has worked and how they have opened the door and got some relief from the rawness of being thrown into this club. The members that have come into the grief club with you all have the possibility of helping each other out of it, like being in an escape room. Working together, not against each other, is the way to achieve this; listening, respecting, and sometimes using each other's techniques to be set free so that the grief club brings peace and comfort rather than pain and despair.

Rachael's Story

Aftermath – Grieving is too difficult.

"What's the point of it all?" Mum had started asking regularly when my sister died suddenly of a brain haemorrhage.

Dad said only this: "The wind has gone out of my sails."

He couldn't say much more than that, and he totally shut down.

The fact is, we were all lost at sea, cast adrift, with no map and no ability to navigate or make sense of what had happened to us.

When Rebecca died, my only sibling, it felt like I lost my past and my future. Our shared life as a family exploded. Our whole sense of who we thought we were as a mother, father and sister seemed to disappear instantly.

Grieving is too difficult; it is all-consuming, unrelenting, and tortuous; it is almost impossible to breathe. Each day is the same as another, as the reality of loss and pain seeps into every part of your mind and body. Initially, it's impossible to understand that the waking nightmare worsens before it gets better. The 'what ifs' and the 'if onlys' arrive hourly throughout the day and night, preventing proper thoughts and sleep. There's a flatness to life so that every normal thing throughout the day feels like you're dragging a lead weight, and no one can quite see or understand how heavy it is.

One morning, probably nine months or so after Rebecca's sudden death, I remember lying in bed listening to the radio. For a moment, I noticed I didn't feel so heavy and that I wasn't consumed by sadness. I listened to and enjoyed the music ("One Day Like This" by Elbow) on the radio. It probably only lasted half an hour, but it gave me hope for the future, a glimmer of the possibility that we could get through this. That's when I started thinking about 'living it double'; if my sister couldn't be here to enjoy her life, I would live it for her.

Seven years later.

Beeeeeeeep... "Stupid woman," I heard a voice shout.

"Oh my god, it's Rachael! Are you okay?"

I'd been walking into the middle of the road, in the village where Mum and Dad lived, oblivious to the traffic, deep in thought. I muttered something about Mum being ill but remembered that this is where I was standing last year when Mum said, "You might as well have my car because I can't drive while I'm on morphine."

A few months later, my Mum died of bowel cancer. We were expecting it, and she passed away in her sleep in the early hours of a Monday morning. It was peaceful, and she was ready. How can you be 'ready' at just sixty-nine years old? She had never regained her joy for life since losing Rebecca.

I'd been here before; I knew that feeling of my body being in one place but my mind being elsewhere - not simply one or two moments of absent-mindedness, but years of it. I'd watched Mum slowly fade away. Had it really been just two years since we went on a trip to Venice together commemorating what would have been Rebecca's fortieth birthday? It felt like both a lifetime and a moment ago, all in the same instant.

I'd started grieving for Mum many years before her actual death so initially it didn't seem real. I couldn't feel it. I was numb. I knew from experience 'that life must go on', and she had told me in no uncertain terms just a few months earlier, "You're forty-six, Rachael; you can look after yourself".

I can still hear her voice saying it, and it makes me smile because she was right! Grief is like a volume fader with someone or something else controlling it. It was a few years after she had gone that I felt the full force of the loss of Mum. I realised that I put a wall up and had been blocking out my feelings, so my mental health was suffering, and I knew I needed help. I don't think I began to grieve for Mum until Dad died eight years later. The finality of losing them all began, and the cumulative grief that followed forced me down a different emotional and psychological path. It's a journey that I'm still on and still learning about. Through it all, there is a way forward and hope!

CHAPTER NINE

WHAT DOES NORMAL MEAN?

It always amazes me how life continues after someone passes when you want to scream at the world to stop. How can this be my new normal when my world is anything but now I have lost a loved one?

The first time I realised this was when I lost my own mother and was feeling the depths of grief physically and mentally. I was sitting by the window in my house, and someone walked by. A surge of anger ran through me like a lightning bolt. I remember thinking about the harsh reality of how the world and life continue despite our pain, expecting us to just carry on as usual, doing normal daily things like shopping, going to work, cleaning and carrying on.

Life continues, but our pain is there locked in our heads, trying to find a way to be dealt with when all around seems to go back to normal, and we feel anything but normal. This can sometimes happen to us abruptly when we lose a loved one. There's the funeral to plan, routines change, people are around having time off work to support each other, and friends check in. Sometimes, it can feel a shock as the first time we find ourselves alone. Suddenly, we have our thoughts to deal with and really feel as though our grieving process has begun.

When the support system that seems to come from nowhere that is in place immediately after a person passes away, while the funeral is being arranged for you, people are checking in on you or when you are busy doing these things yourself, the moment then hits you when normal life resumes a life to us that will never be the same again. This is where we must dig deep, take care of ourselves, and begin to take control of the grief that is now part of our new normal.

To start a new journey, we must start over and try to rediscover and find ourselves so that we can feel the joy once again that was lost in the early days of the grieving process, and that can constantly rob us of those moments.

Depending on the stage you are at in your life, sometimes it's almost like you haven't got time to grieve. Having young children, while challenging, tends to provide us with structure as they need it, sometimes making it seem easier as we don't have to work out our new routine. We may have to return to work for financial reasons, but we don't know how to cope. We sometimes must make the effort ourselves; it is a hard lesson to learn and takes a lot of courage. Having a life that has a healthy routine helps us to grieve healthily; keeping to a regular sleep pattern and eating regular meals will all help you heal. Engaging with others, doing new things, and picking up the telephone to call someone are all ways to help us not feel so isolated.

The new normal can feel overwhelming at first, but in time, it will become the normal. Set yourself goals like always making sure you speak to another person if you live alone. On the flip side, if you are around people all day, make sure you take some time out during that day to be able to feel and process your thoughts.

Harry's Story

Grief is one of the toughest things that anyone could go through. It changes you and makes you think of strange thoughts and decisions. Losing someone, no matter who it is, whether it be a pet, family or friend, all feels the same. Losing three members was hard for me, especially since they all happened within a year; I would have never thought I would have been able to handle it, but here I am, defeating the grief and battling on, and that's all we can do!

During the whole grief stage, I found it helpful to sit back and watch how different people deal with it and to try someone else's methods on yourself until you find which suits you. I found keeping busy and doing the things they would have wanted you to do helps instead of doing nothing and getting lost in your thoughts. Talking, working, doing hobbies, anything at all, just keeping the mind busy, taking each day as it comes, and never quitting - that helped me!

But before any of my doing, I learnt all this from my amazing family, who supported me through thick and thin. They have been there at dark times and brighter times. They kept me going when I wanted to quit and when I thought things were over, and they taught me valuable lessons on handling it! Family is so important, and it's always nice to know you have someone there. Dealing with grief alone is one of the hardest things I have dealt with. A quick chat or a little trip out of the house with someone always changes my mood. All these lessons have taught me to feel comfortable helping others in the same situation. The human body is a strange, wonderful, crazy thing. We all feel different; listening to other's stories is so important. It helped me a lot.

Some days, I feel like crying; some days, I feel like cheering, but no matter what, keep going for the ones we have lost and keep going for yourself. They played their amazing part, and now it's time for us to carry it on! They are always with you, no matter what. My amazing family got me through my grief, and I couldn't be more thankful.

CHAPTER TEN

INTRUSIVE THOUGHTS

The thoughts and feelings that flood our brains during grieving can, at times, feel out of control. We normally go about our day before grief, thinking about what we may do, planning social events, sleeping, working, etc. Grief has no respect for the order of normal life.

Unfortunately, although we already have enough to deal with grieving and all that entails about the loved one we have lost, it can bring along other unwanted thoughts and emotions we have to deal with. Here is another scenario, like a slap in the face.

I remember having a whole week of anxiety and intrusive thoughts. I had to keep talking myself around because I feared what would happen next and who would be the next person I would lose. Tons of questions flooded my mind, scrambling about, and then I realised there were no answers to these intrusive, unwanted thoughts.

We must return to what we preach to ourselves, what we know is best for us and our wellbeing. We must be present now to enjoy this moment, knowing the past can't be changed and that it's impossible to know our future. When we master this technique, we open up a whole new pathway for ourselves. Of course, it takes time, and we fall off the path and must reset and remember to be kind to ourselves.

The thoughts will come into your brain like an unwanted intruder walking straight into your house. Then they sit in your brain while we work out what to do with them - waiting to be entertained and torturing and disrupting our wellbeing, peace, and structure of our usual life. We have no choice but to deal with it. Sometimes, we feel completely overwhelmed by these new thoughts, tired and drained, and hopeless, having to constantly deal with these intruders in our heads. We want to sleep to rest and avoid dealing with it at that moment.

One thing about the grieving thoughts is that they come and go. When you have thoughts that are particularly painful and hard to deal with, flying in from nowhere, and feeling in a dark place, you must remember to tell yourself that these thoughts will pass. A different one will step in its place. We must work through feelings and emotions from grieving. Still, unhelpful intrusive thoughts require a different strategy in that we must let them go so as not to interfere with the natural grieving process, as it is unhelpful and damaging to our delicate grieving mind.

We can sit in the same chair on a different week and feel different, in a completely different head space. So, remember whatever that thought is, we can sit in the same chair again with a totally different mindset as it will pass. Gain strength in that and use it as a mantra for yourself. *This feeling will pass. I will sit here in the same space again and again, knowing I can be in a different place in my mind. The struggling thoughts will pass.*

Distraction is one way of changing these unwanted thoughts. Do something to take your mind away from them. You are not your thoughts; you are more than this. They will go.

Change your thought pattern. If you keep getting a reoccurring one, and you feel you have dealt with it, but it keeps giving you a hard time, replace it with a positive one or a nice memory you have.

We will also develop our own skills in ways to lose these thoughts, to help us cope. It is normal to feel like this as part of a grieving process, and this is why, in the early days, we must give ourselves time to protect ourselves and learn how we will react to provide us with the confidence to move forward. When feeling a little stronger, your inner strength will amaze you, coming through when needed. You may have to dig deep to find it, but it's there waiting for you to pull it out and work through the emotions forced upon you when grieving.

As always, if you aren't managing your thoughts and it is impacting your daily life so you cannot function, ask for help to manage your symptoms. Your GP can refer you for this.

Tamzin's Story

Age 20

Grief is not something I ever encountered to be as hard as it is. It's a whirlwind of mixed emotions, some visible and some we all keep hidden and deep underneath our skin.

Grief, for me, was a handful of physical and emotional thoughts and feelings. My first symptom of grief was sadness and an overwhelming cloud that still, to this day, I cannot shift. I continually asked myself what I could have done better. Could I have done this better? Why me? And most importantly, why them?

I found myself alone with my thoughts, which started a war for myself and others. Grief had made me so numb I couldn't see who I was hurting and how I was hurting myself, with all these dark thoughts plummeting around my mind. I remember endlessly and randomly flooding with tears with anything I could relate back at that moment as sentimental value to my loved one. Butterflies and buckets of adrenaline overran my mind and body. Shortly after this I became angry and confused to why

I was crying at the smallest thing I could usually deal with before losing a loved one. Many things could easily trigger this war, such as a location, a smell or a piece of clothing - things that my mind had screenshotted and placed into a core memory to remember them by.

My grief still lingers over me daily. I try to shut it out, but these dark thoughts seem to be never-ending. I try to occupy my mind with things I love, keep myself busy, and not be defeated to sit and dwell on these emotions. Some days I can barely move from one place. My motivation drains from me, and all I can think about is how much pain I am feeling from within. These emotions and feelings can sometimes stop me from doing things I enjoy, which saddens me even more. When will this end? Nighttime for me is the worst as my mind loves to dig deep into days, weeks and years from the past, and I cannot switch off and get overfilled with guilt, worry and anxiety.

However, I know each day is a new day, each year is a new chapter, and from my loved one passing, I only want to make them proud to keep the fire lit as they did when they lost their loved ones. I think to myself they carried on for us so we should do the same for them. And each day, when the dark thoughts drift over, I push them back, and I get up and challenge them.

As someone wise once told me, "Depression is your body's way of saying it's not happy with the life you're living." Since that day, I remind myself that it's okay to be sad. You're only human, but never let the fear inside beat you. Because I know I was raised strong, and if I could be half as strong as they were, I know I have won. And I now look at grief not so much as a bad thing but as this - grief is the final goodbye to our loved one. It's remembering how much we loved them and, most importantly, how much they loved you. In a way, it reflects every small detail of that person, from a scent to a place to even maybe a "random" thing. It is your body's way of sending back their presents and love.

WHAT AM I STRUGGLING WITH?

CHAPTER ELEVEN

TRIGGERS

What defines a trigger is an intense and usually negative emotion.

I have found over the years and going through different grieving processes, triggers come in many forms, shapes and sizes. Some obvious ones affect us, like hearing a song that reminds us of a special someone we have lost; I have found that sometimes the little personal ones can catch you unaware.

Dealing with triggers is a constant battle in the early days. They can appear from nowhere, forcing us to deal with them there and then, and we must face them and feel them to work through them. If we don't allow ourselves this feeling it brings on, we will store it in our heads and must deal with an overload of unworked triggers, which is too much to cope with.

As we work through the triggers and the emotion it carries with it, we will then recognise them in the future without them completely freaking us out. We will become one with them; ultimately, this is the goal. Allowing ourselves to feel inner peace takes time, and we must work our way towards this. After the healing process of grief, some of them will turn into beautiful memories that can actually bring you joy instead of pain. It's impossible to see this in the early stage of grieving. It will happen only when we have had time to digest our triggers and work through them.

Triggers link us to the person we loved and lost. I remember going into town just before Christmas, after my mother passed, and crying over brussels sprouts because of a childhood memory of my mum sitting there peeling piles of them and being overwhelmed with sadness. Brussels sprouts had triggered me! It was the fact she couldn't be here for any more of my Christmases. These triggers are powerful and can come at any time. They are all personal and unique to us because of our own personal experiences.

Triggers are charged with emotion; they can come at us like a lightning bolt when we least expect it; triggers will keep happening in many scenarios throughout our lives, missing the person we have lost. As time goes on and we have no choice but to move forward in our grief, we can work towards them not feeling so painful. Unfortunately, this is ongoing in the grief world, forming a part of our new life. One strategy is to be in the triggering scenario and make them proud as if you were doing your best.

Grieving is tiring as we must constantly work through the sadness of all the thoughts and triggers being thrown at us, wading through until a day comes when we can look at what was once a trigger as a memory we can cherish. I promise you this will come, but not without doing the grieving homework.

We will slip back and react in a way that is not how we want again. Work through it, note how it makes you feel, and think about how you would have liked to react. Please don't be hard on yourself. It's a process that takes time to get to where we want to be. We must give ourselves the space and thinking time to go through the process of recognition. By working on them, we can react in a way we feel at ease with, a feeling of safety within our own thoughts, and feel in control when this happens. It's not easy when a trigger happens and a reaction of, let's say, anger comes out; we say things we don't mean to, which can snowball into more grief and upset, but we can recharge and move on from these negative responses to help us react in a way we are happy with.

When we first lose someone, it is important to give ourselves time and space to process the loss. Be kind to yourself during this time. We are amazing at assessing ourselves, so listen to your gut and do what's right for you.

Chelsie's Story

Age 32

There isn't a day you don't enter my mind. Sometimes, they are good thoughts, and sometimes, they are thoughts I wish you never would put there.

I try to make them go away, but it's so difficult sometimes. I have so many happy memories with you, but sometimes they get overtaken by a feeling I don't think will ever go away. Grief is horrible, let alone when you don't have the answers you need, and it can consume you on the bad days.

Sometimes I don't want to think about you so I can try to be normal and not think about why you are not here anymore, then I feel guilty for thinking like that. I know I am not the only one who is going through this. Sometimes, you must let it out - AND TALK.

My heart goes out to anyone that has lost someone too and is feeling this way. I just wish you never left this world. Miss you forever, KB.

MY GRIEF TRIGGERS ARE...

CHAPTER TWELVE

GRIEF AND ADDICTION

What is addiction? It means you are addicted to something that, in turn, is causing you harm.

It can be described as the intense urge to use a substance that's addictive or behaves in a certain way that will harm you and have negative consequences. Drugs and alcohol change the state of mind.

It's extremely difficult to grieve healthily while having an addiction. Being dependent is having an addiction.

I have worked with many people with addictions over the years. One thing that always stayed with me throughout this and being able to empathise and help others is that no one set out to be an addict. The pull of the addiction is immense, robbing people of their personality, families, homes and lives. Some people manage their addiction well, and then a situation like losing a loved one can send it spiralling out of control. Most have started off casually and, for a host of different reasons, found themselves hooked, not in control, and unable to stop.

One of the reasons I would hear time and time again is that a person's addiction was to numb pain, a way of initially dealing with their emotions, not to have to feel them, to mask them and feel as though all is okay. This, of course, is only temporary; when the feeling of alcohol or drugs has worn off, the pain is still there, along with a hangover or comedown, adding to the sense of pain and distress, and the cycle starts again.

You are depleting your energy to deal with the real problem, affecting your sleep and strength, and you are in a cycle of addiction. Using substances can delay the reaction of grief, so it still must be unpacked even years after losing someone. Hidden feelings and emotions with minds clouded with substances and addictions stop us from grieving naturally, working through our feelings, and being able to live a life after grief. It's impossible to hide from grief; it can feel as though you can delay it, you have escaped it, but it will always, without doubt, must be worked through. There is no escaping it by using other means.

With the right help and support, it's possible to become free of addiction and become free of the grief that's been hiding behind it. You don't have to try and overcome this alone, and you're entitled to NHS health care to help with this. A good starting point is your GP. There are specific places to get help for drug and alcohol use and any other type of addiction you may have; find out where your local service is to get support. Support groups are amazing sources of help at this time. To be surrounded by people who have been and understand where you're at is invaluable, and it's a blessing to not feel alone. They can support you to rebuild your life without addiction.

You deserve to get your life back and be free from addiction; being able to cope and grieve while being supported will be vital for your wellbeing during this time.

With the right help and support it's possible to become free of addiction and become free of the grief that's been hiding behind it.

Lynsay's Poem

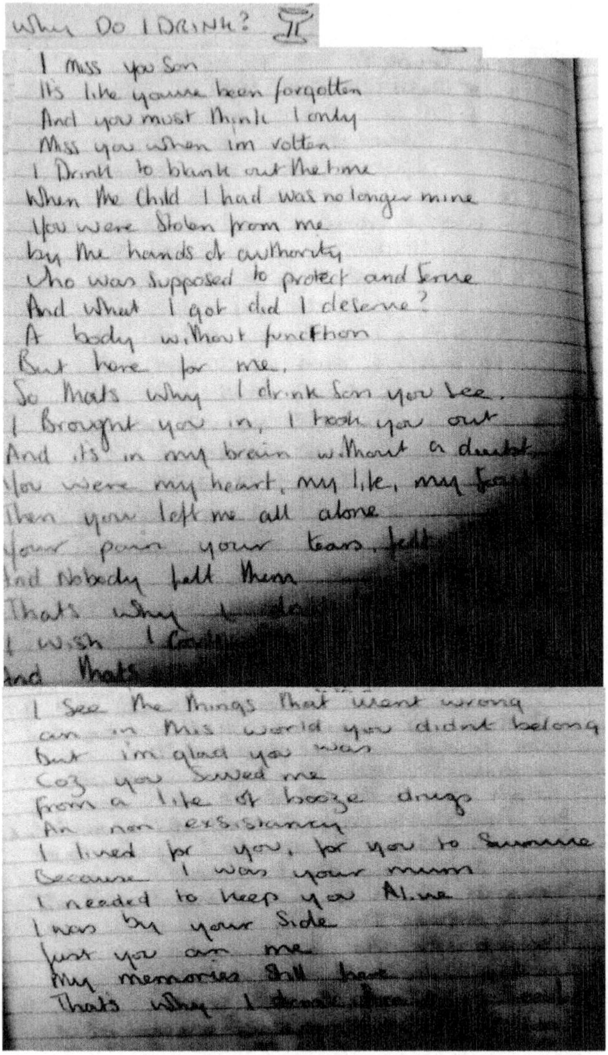
Why Do I Drink?
I miss you Son
It's like you've been forgotten
And you must think I only
Miss you when im rotten
I Drink to blank out the time
When the Child I had was no longer mine
You were Stolen from me
by the hands of authority
Who was supposed to protect and Serve
And what I got did I deserve?
A body without function
But here for me.
So thats why I drink Son you see.
I brought you in, I took you out
And its in my brain without a doubt
You were my heart, my life, my [illegible]
Then your left me all alone
Your pain your tears fell
And Nobody felt them
Thats why I [illegible]
I wish I Could [illegible]
And thats [illegible]
I see the things that went wrong
an in this world you didnt belong
But im glad you was
Coz you Saved me
from a life of booze drugs
An non exsistancy
I lived for you, for you to Survive
Because I was your mum
I needed to keep you Alive
I was by your Side
Just you an me
My memories Still here
Thats why I [illegible]

SOMETHING THAT HAS HELPED ME COPE TODAY?

CHAPTER THIRTEEN

LOVE HURTS

Without love, there is no grief.

We are grieving because we have loved; our pain is intense because this love has been our world. Love takes time and gets deeper. Our worlds have been entwined because of our love and care for this person. It has created beautiful memories for us.

Love is made up of many little things, making everything feel different. We crave that the person be here, but the love they gave us is still with us and still in our hearts.

Through our grieving, we find the love we shared a comfort - a precious part of life when they were here that no one can destroy or take away from us. It remains locked in the safety of our hearts so we can feel it as a comfort once again. The love with the person we have lost has kept us going on many occasions while they were alive. Sit with this thought and remember how that love made us feel, and, more importantly, remember that love is still in us. It hasn't gone away.

While working through our emotions, we seek the grief to live peacefully alongside the love we were lucky to have, to gain strength from it and the positives this love brought to us. In time, it helps us heal.

Without love, there is no grief.

Georgie-Leigh

Age: 12

What Greif means to me:
When a loved one passes it makes me feel incredibly upset. The reason I feel this way is the thought of never seeing them again. I also had moments of happiness for remembering all of the fun and happy memories we have together. Something that helped me get through this point in time is talking to people around you. Also keeping your head up and thinking of the happy memmories. Just remember, when your in the darkness always look for light! :)!!

CHAPTER FOURTEEN

SUICIDE GRIEF

The grieving of someone taking their own life feels different, like grief on steroids. Ultimately, the result is the same: we no longer have the person we love with us, but it feels heavier, deeper, intense, and complicated as we try and wrap our heads around the loss and the big 'why'. It sends our brains into a completely different process as usually, when we die, the choice of living is taken away from us.

When someone makes that choice to leave us in this world and not be here, it opens a whole new world of a tangled web of new emotions you never knew were there. This is when I found out this type of grieving is called complex grief, which says it in a nutshell, and I got it: a whole new load of stuff to wade through like nothing you have ever dealt with before. You may look for an answer that may come to some, believing that it then brings the individual who has passed peace after they have lived a painful or chaotic life.

I believe that the start of this process is not to torture yourself with the what-ifs, the questions we will never know the answer to. We must grieve for the person we know, not send ourselves into a spiral of complete despair trying to find answers but find some peace to move forward into a life that will never be the same again. We must remember all our beautiful memories and not lose them in the complexity of unanswered questions.

I have read that people who took their own lives do so as they feel it's the only way to get out of how they are feeling. They don't want to die but feel there is no alternative to their thoughts and the pain and hopelessness they are feeling. We must remove the torment and guilt from ourselves to allow ourselves to heal. 'Peace after pain' were the words my daughter said to me a year after her husband had passed away. I wanted to find more peace this year, so I felt her words. We continue to walk on this path and work towards this.

Losing someone to suicide feels very different from losing a loved one, where the choice is out of their control. It creates a sense of loss like no other. A time of uncertainty and fear awaits us amongst the complexity of this. A world you knew changed dramatically, and the remains feel embedded in you, a forever process of dealing with life. It helps to take one day, sometimes one hour or even one minute at a time, to keep moving forward, being aware that, good or bad, nothing stays the same.

I had previously spent time trying to live mindfully, to appreciate every day, and to be in the present moment. I realised that losing my son-in-law in this way had catapulted me into a place of living for the here and now, as we never know what tomorrow will bring. It was like this was my only hope and all I had to cling to as it was my only coping strategy, and it worked. So, in the madness of my thoughts, I try to ground myself in all that I have today, be truly grateful for that, and live in the now and focus on what is happening.

Being present and not focusing on negative pasts or worrying about an uncertain future is far more helpful than a future worry that may never happen, as is being thankful for today and trying to live positively, even though the tough emotions of grief keep coming up like a punch in the face to deal with. This must be a good enough reason to live for today and be grateful for all the good you have in your life in this present moment.

MY STORY

My daughter Chloe met my son-in-law Kyle when they were fourteen, and they were inseparable from that day. They made us proud by buying a house, getting engaged, then married, and having two beautiful sons. They loved the boys and each other unconditionally.

It was a normal day. I was preparing dinner and waiting for my husband and son to come home when my daughter rang to say my six-year-old grandson had a haircut; he always went with his Dad. She had spoken to her husband earlier that day to check the arrangements and had a normal conversation. She said he hadn't come home from work, and the first reaction was that there would be a simple answer. However, he never let anyone down and was always ready to help someone, so it was totally out of his character. She knew where he was working, so she went with my husband, leaving my two grandsons, aged six and nine months old, with me. She thought he may have had an accident as he was a plasterer working alone in a house with no stairs. I wondered if he had chipped off to help someone, given them a lift, and left his phone behind.

My daughter called me to say his van was locked up outside the house. I thought this was typical of my thinking, which is why he wasn't answering. Then, my son came home from work. We were in the business that dinner time brings with my grandsons, laughing and playing, and all of us were in our safe world.

Elsewhere, my husband broke into the house, as it was locked, to double-check that my son-in-law hadn't fallen and had an accident.

We were all blissfully unaware of the devastation to come.

My husband discovered my son-in-law inside and that he had taken his own life. With my daughter waiting outside, my husband had to go and tell her what had happened. At that moment, all our lives, his wife, their children, his brothers, Mum and Dad, family and friends changed forever, throwing us all into a cycle of complex grief.

Due to the shock, we were still naively unaware of the type of grief that was to come and what we all had to deal with and still now constantly deal with.

My son, my grandsons, and I were in our home. Everything was the same, but all had changed. None of our lives would be the same again. The next hour of thought is still patchy, as there is no sense to be made of what had happened. I know we were deeply shocked, and it was painful. I remember us just walking around, holding our heads at one point in disbelief, not being able to take in the devastation of it all.

We rang my other daughter, who was at work, and told her what had happened. She came and took the boys home with my granddaughter and kept them for the night. I remember being comforted by the fact that she had brought them home as I looked at them. I was grateful they didn't know and could be in their home for a night without knowing what had happened. I was relieved knowing they were safe, still being shielded from how their lives would be affected forever.

My daughter came back with my husband, and her face had changed so much that I hardly recognised her. Her expression, full of pain and shock, will haunt me forever. As her mum, this was the first time I knew I couldn't take her pain away. It was devastating.

I had to ring my son-in-law's Mum and Dad, making it the worst phone call ever; within what seemed like seconds, his close family and ours, all together, were in shock, reeling from deep feelings of pain, despair, disbelief, tears and overwhelmed with 'why'. We all sat in a room full of family that loved him, and he loved in return.

It was then our journey of grieving started. It is nearly impossible to write what this entails. From that moment, your whole life has changed; everything about your mind that comforted you has gone, leaving you with pure tormented grief.

Everyone left my home; I did not know how long everyone had been there. My husband and son eventually went to bed, leaving my daughter and me downstairs. We were up all night. Our main conversation was about how we would tell his sons - he loved them all so much. It was something a mother should never have to do, and we had no idea how.

We started to google ways to help us as we were afraid of wrongly explaining it and hurting them even more, which weighed heavily on us. Every thought of them was like a knife stabbing our hearts.

We came across the charity Winston's Wish. They support children through grief, help them process it, and support them to find ways to move forward for a brighter future. However, they were closed at that time. We planned to ring them in the morning to get some advice.

We rang them as soon as it opened; they were kind and supportive and explained the best way to tell them at six and nine months old. One whose world would change forever, whom we could talk to, and the other younger child we could encourage to communicate how he felt. They also sent out a big pack of information to help, books for the children, ways to deal with questions they ask - not only now but at all the different ages, with advice of appropriate wording and language for them to be able to understand and process. All this was a great help in guiding us from experts who knew how to help. It relieved us and helped us to know they had clarified what to say so we did not add to their pain.

My daughter told her son, which was the hardest thing she has ever had to do. Children are resilient and amazing; we have always found to answer their questions age appropriately as it comforts them, and they are then satisfied for that moment. If another question arises, answer it again with lots of love, support, and communication. The experts assured us they would be okay.

I have often said I want to be able to grieve as a child does, as we can be our own worst enemies in our own minds and thoughts. I have learnt that one way a child can achieve this is by living in the moment, the here and now. When we do this as adults, it helps, as I've discovered. Of course, it takes time to be more mindful, but we can do it.

I only learnt about complex grief when my son-in-law took his own life. I feel so sad for what he must have been going through himself, and for us all, we had no warning or reason for this to happen. Losing someone you love this way is extremely hard to describe; it is so traumatic. So, the shock and disbelief you feel when you find this out is immense, and your brain is not wired to take in such horrific news. Working your way through intense feelings, emotions, and confusion is ongoing. I miss him so much. We are doing our best, and we are extremely blessed to have beautiful children to love.

I beg anyone with any suicidal thoughts to speak up. Whatever the situation, your life is always worth it; feelings will change and feel different. Seek help, as there is always a way to feel different.

The SAMARITANS is a helpline where you can confidentially talk to someone if you are struggling. It has a twenty-four-hour telephone line. The telephone number is 116 123, and it is free to call from any phone.

When your brain starts to thaw out from the initial shock of always having to live with constant moments of disbelief, then to be thrown into beginning the grieving process is where the complexity comes in; one of the biggest challenges to deal with is that it was their choice, which is overwhelming to deal with. I find thinking of my son-in-law and how he loved his family up to just before he passed away comforting. It can help ease off from torturing yourself with questions we will never know the answers to; of course, that is a battle, but one thing I have learnt along the way is that constant questioning brings more pain.

Losing someone to suicide feels like the acceptance part of the grieving cycle has been removed, leaving you in a heightened state of grief to constantly deal with it. It requires you to find a totally different way of thinking and to be able to manage your life.

Sometimes, without any knowledge of the person you have lost, some think it's okay to voice their opinion to you. They have no idea what you're going through and how unkind this is. We must learn quickly not to take those negative opinions on board. Remember the person you loved and the love they had for you, and do not be concerned about others' opinions.

I've learnt through this loss that although we are grieving, and of course the same emotions occur as losing someone to natural causes, it throws a lot more at you to deal with. There's a turmoil of emotions, and each one feels intensified. You do not know where to go with them or how to deal with them alongside the grief, shock, and desperation of missing the person you loved, seeing your loved ones hurting with no answers, and thoughts of what to tell the children when they ask a question. It's a case of battling through this new way of living by fighting through a terrifying barrier of thoughts every day to keep going.

As we wear our grief mask of coping, we know it must come off to overcome some of our grief to work through it. We aim to understand our triggers, to try and live again with the inner peace we crave, to function without pain and to live our lives knowing it will never be or feel the same again. Complex grief is hard to explain, as constant, complicated grief doesn't leave you much clear head space to work with.

It's been a year since we lost my amazing son-in-law, so we have now done all the grieving firsts. These are painful: birthdays, Christmas, anniversaries, etc, when you long for them to be with you all again. We've had to try to bring back and focus on some of the happiness we felt when he was here to feel as we did while also knowing it will never be the same. As we work through the tough days, we know no one can take our beautiful memories away. Thinking of the person we've lost as if they have just moved on before us to the next room while we are still here is the job of a lifetime. We will always be trying to master and learn how to get through, knowing our bad days will always come while we look for a ray of light up to the stars to help us.

We are lucky that we are all close - our family and my son-in law's family and friends have all supported each other. This has been such a large part of recovery for us and magnifies how important it is to communicate with each other. Not everyone has this, so finding a way to express yourself is important. To help heal, writing down your thoughts about what you would say to the loved one you lost can help to release them and any attached emotions from your mind about what you never got a chance to say. You can write a one-off letter, write daily thoughts, or just write when your head feels full.

SOBS - Survivors of Bereavement by Suicide is a support group that holds meetings locally in lots of different towns and cities to support people. I found them by searching for help on the internet. They are amazing; they have a support line with people to talk to and it will save you if you feel like you need some help in processing your grief.

Whether it's through therapy, talking to friends or support groups, it's not a process to go through alone. There is help. Speak to your doctor or get a friend to do it with you if you don't feel able. The strength you gain through support from people you know truly understand is important in dealing with complex grief. To help heal some of the pain, be gentle on yourself and do it day by day.

We are still trying to heal as a family and run our lives along the grief we are all experiencing. The children have helped us with the joy and laughter they bring. I am so lucky to have a daughter who is an amazing Mum whose strength has been outstanding; she is an inspiration, keeping their amazing Dad's memory alive and helping the boys to live a happy life. We all walk alongside each other in this together, and my advice is that communication makes you feel less alone in all of this; talking to each other helps ease some of the pain. All his family and ours still help carry each other along in times of need and will always be doing this to keep moving forward. For this, I'm truly grateful.

WHAT SUPPORT DO I HAVE WHILE GRIEVING?

CHAPTER FIFTEEN

GRIEF AND ITS HORRIBLE GRIEF FRIENDS

Losing someone we love is a unique experience for us. My relationship with the person who passed is different from yours, but we travel together on the grieving journey. Sometimes, this journey runs smoothly, and we can make sense of some of our feelings. Other times, it's like a train speeding along, and we can't get off with our emotions whizzing around in our heads, yearning for some peace.

We look the same from the outside, but the inside is broken. We must set aside time to try and work through these thoughts, unravel them, and piece together our new world to allow us to move forward on our journey. It is a journey which can be peaceful once again with a head that can think clearly again, that is not having a conversation about one thing with other thoughts constantly about the person we have lost dancing around at the back of our mind so we can't think straight. We must try and fix ourselves, and this pattern is exhausting.

In the early days of grieving and when the grief wave comes and goes, we must travel it with all the trauma it brings. We know where the journey began but don't know where it will end.

I learnt there are different types of grief, a whole horrible grief family all related to each other, leaving us with a whole lot to cope with, which can make our journey a lot rockier. I always thought that if someone passed away, we would all feel the same, but that's impossible as I am me, and you are you. Also, we must consider how someone passes, their age, and the complex relationship we have with them all have a big impact on our grieving process. Not only is it always hard, but the circumstances can bring different pain and emotions to work through. We are all unique beings, so we must navigate our own journey. Now, what's right for one may not be suitable for another, but that's okay. We are like pilots flying a plane without a license, not knowing how we will land. We go through the black clouds and wait for the lighter ones to appear to feel lifted again, to drop out of nowhere when we hit turbulence like our minds pulled in and out of states of grief scrambling around to find our new pathway out of the pain to feel free again and find peace.

Here are some types of grief, showing how unique our experiences are and how much we must deal with, magnifying the importance of dealing with it. Grief must be felt and dealt with to come through it.

Distorted grief

An extreme reaction, like anger, often characterises this. Distorted grief provokes an intense emotional response, which one can direct at others or at oneself.

Chronic or complicated grief

This is when the usual pattern of grieving we work through intensifies over time instead of subsiding.

Delayed grief

When the normal pattern of grieving doesn't occur as expected, a reaction to grief occurs later than usual.

Masked grief

This is a symptom of grief in which you are not saying you have or are hiding; you are masking your feelings.

Exaggerated grief

In this instance, one experiences more intense reactions like suicidal thoughts or self-destructive behaviours to cope with the feelings of grief through substance misuse, drugs and alcohol.

Anticipatory grief

These are feelings of grief or loss before we lose the person. This is common if someone has a terminal illness.

Persistent and prolonged grief

This is intense, prolonged grief that causes problems daily in your life. Grieving is a natural response; for most of us, it does get better with time.

Complex grief

With this type, there is an extreme focus on the person's death, an intense longing and pining for your loss, feeling a sense of loss on your purpose in life, and obsessively thinking about your grief constantly.

When you look at the stages and types of grief we must complete to come through it, it's easy to see why it's so hard and the toll it takes on us physically and mentally. Listen to your body and mind as life throws us into this cycle. It is normal to be in any of these states of mind while grieving and dependent on your circumstances.

Grief is there to work through; it shouldn't be your whole life and existence forever, stopping your life and thoughts of other things. Of course, in the early days of losing someone, this is what happens, but you will keep moving through your grief.

If you feel stuck, unable to keep moving with it and continuing with your life, eventually finding moments of hope, light, and little bursts of happiness and peace, and feeling like you are on the right side of grief, you may need help to move forward. Grief has no timeline sometimes but keep checking in on yourself that it isn't dark all the time and that moments of light do eventually keep appearing.

CHLOE'S STORY

AGE 34

When I lost my husband, my whole world collapsed around me. I can remember in detail what I did that day up until I found out he had died.

After that, the next few weeks are a total blur. I was so numb; I couldn't focus, I couldn't feel, I couldn't process conversations, I didn't know what day or time it was, and I had all the anxiety symptoms but with no anxious thoughts.

When the feelings did come, I had no idea how big these emotions would be. They totally consumed me - all of them: sadness, anger, hopelessness, guilt and fear. A lot of the time, when the feelings did get too consuming, my brain would automatically switch to numbness; I think it was my mind protecting me from spiralling too far.

Grief has changed me: the way I think, the way I eat, the way I look and the way I parent.

One of my earliest memories after my husband died was being in a supermarket for the first time and looking around at everyone just going about their day as normal, thinking, how can everything around me be so normal when my world is falling apart?

In the early days of loss, people would tell me how strong I was, and that time was a healer. I know people mean well when they say these things, but I still don't believe them to be true. I am not strong; I have no choice. Time is not a healer; I just must learn how to live with the fact that I will miss him forever.

What I have learned over the last twelve months is that I can't look forward anymore because, to me, it is still unimaginable to have a future without him in it. So, I look backwards to see how far I have come and what I have achieved. Things I could never imagine doing again, like the school run, making dinner, going out with friends, going on holiday, laughing and returning to work. I must look backwards to keep moving forwards.

WHAT AM I FEARFUL OF FACING?

CHAPTER SIXTEEN

THE STILLNESS OF GRIEF

Grieving is hard work. And some days, it's okay to give in to it. If time allows, go with it; permit yourself to sit with or without feelings. You don't have to be strong and okay - you can sit in the stillness of grief. It recharges us through grieving and rests our minds while sitting and staring into space. Release the need to function, communicate, watch television, or scroll through social media - you can shut yourself off from the world.

When these days come, you can embrace them, sitting as if time has stopped. Just know that these days often come out of the blue, but they also do pass. You know you could pick up the phone or go out, but nothing needs to happen when you are paralysed with grief and need just to be still. We will understand these days are necessary, as it's nature's way of allowing us to heal. They are different from being depressed. If we spent day after day for weeks like this, we would be stuck in a grief phase. We might then realise we need to talk to someone, be kind to ourselves and get the help we need if we feel unable to push through it.

Claire's story

I was thirty-six when I lost my 'Big' Nana, who, at the grand old age of ninety-three, had most definitely had a good innings! I had only ever lost my 'Little Nana' before that. Being eleven when that happened, I remember laughing (from embarrassment as my family told me the news), then crying bucketloads, and then not shedding another tear ever again in my life; so, when I lost Big Nana, it's fair to say I had never experienced proper grief before. (Disclaimer: one Nana was shorter than the other; they didn't pitch against each other in a weight comparison war, and if they were ever offended by my monikers for them, they were good enough Nana's not to show it!)

Of course, I'd known people I cared about die, but my Nana was like a second mum to me - I was the daughter she never had, and I knew it! So, although I should have perhaps been expecting her to go, given her circumstances of cancer on top of her grand old age, I stupidly thought she would live forever! And I thought she had been doing an excellent job of doing just that up until she died!

I remember feeling really, REALLY sad for days and days and days on end after she died. Sadness for her that she was no longer here, sadness for me that she was no longer here and a sadness that crept up on me out of nowhere when I thought I was okay. It was Easter time when she died, and I'll never forget making a cake with my boys and having to stop myself from crying over the bowl of cake batter! I could spend all day thinking about her and not feel sad, and then there it would be, an overwhelming flood of devastation that I would never see her again!

The funny thing about that is that I truly believe I will see her again, and it's because of things she told me that I believe it, but none of that mattered initially when she died. That said, I do think it's that belief that enables me to think about my Nana without feeling sad anymore. I believe that she is back with all her brothers and sisters, her beloved husband and all her good friends. The sad thing about living until you're ninety-three is that you outlive everyone, and my Nana had done just that. The only people she had left on this earth were my Dad, my brother and me, and that's without mentioning the daily pain and confusion she was in. It's quite selfish of me to still want her here with me when considering all that!

I still miss her desperately, of course. We were like two peas in a pod. No one had my corner like she did, not even my parents. The thirty-six-year belief I had that she would always be around still leaves me with disbelief that she isn't sometimes, which is totally irrational and something lodged in my psyche after years of banter with her that she would! She sadly never got to see me get married. Still, I was lucky enough for her to meet both my children, and she doted on them just as much as she had me, if not more so, and for that, I am extremely grateful.

I've been fortunate enough in my life not to have experienced personal grief many times at all. I think I've found other people's grief harder to process, some instances of which have been absolutely hideous and left me feeling not only beyond helpless but, be it rightly or wrongly, more devastated for the living than the dead. With this in mind, it's quite difficult for me to write a passage about the subject because I don't have much experience. I know that it hurts, feels desperate, and almost always comes as a shock, but I also know (and here is where I sound like a mad woman) that I will see those people I love again. Whether that's true or not, who knows? I suppose one day I'll find out!

CHAPTER SEVENTEEN

YOUR INNER STRENGTH

I have often written in a bereavement card to a family member or friend when they have lost someone: 'Your inner strength will come through to guide you when you need it most.' I have experienced this on many occasions when grieving.

This strength will come in its most beneficial forms when you need it most, and sometimes, you may not even realise or recognise it. Think back to how you have dealt with something and got through a part of grieving you have done that you never thought you would - for example, the funeral arrangements and conversating your way through the decisions you must make by having hard conversations. We have found that strength and proved to ourselves that we can. It is important for us to remember how strong we already have been without even realising it. We must remember we can find that inner strength again. It's inside us, and we sometimes must search for it again, reaching deep inside and telling ourselves, 'We have this, and we can get through this.'

We should use our strength to explore and tackle hard times and our feelings instead of trying to get rid of them like a blanket that's suffocating us. By untangling all the feelings, we get to move forward like unravelling a knotted ball of string. It is amazing what we can deal with even when we don't realise it. Sometimes, it will arise when we least expect it, and other times, we must look a little deeper inside ourselves. At some point, your inner strength will come to empower you and guide you. Embrace the positive side of you this brings in moving forward with your grief.

Nicola's story

My Mum passed away at the age of sixty-eight, and to say I was devastated was an understatement. I remember leaving the hospital on the day Mum passed away and felt complete numbness, shock and fear of not having my Mum in my life anymore. Who would be there for you like your Mum is/was? Who would know and love you like your Mum? I remember I sobbed so much and exhausted myself. However, that night, I was petrified to go to sleep as it would mean the reality of waking up in the morning to a new day and the start of many days when I didn't have my Mum.

I was in a blur for the next few weeks, and I asked my sister to come back to the hospital ward where Mum had passed away. I needed closure on the fact my Mum was ready to pass away, and they hadn't got it wrong. Looking back now, I appreciate that it was me in denial, and at the height of my grief, the nurses explained everything to me and made me understand what happens when our bodies shut down.

I knew my world would never be the same again—the first birthday, Christmas, Mother's Day. I dreaded them all and had to tell myself it was just another day, and Mum was around us and always would be. I couldn't look at photos, Mum's clothes, cards, or letters she had written for many months, but in a strange way, I got comfort from having lots of Mum's trinkets on show.

One night, around six months after Mum had passed away, I read a card and a letter Mum had written to me. I lay on my bed and howled with tears and cried and cried. I remember the feeling of never seeing my Mum again or having a phone call from her. Mum used to love buying us cards, bookmarks, and books about daughters, and I have kept every single one. So, I feel very lucky I have all these memories and Mum's handwriting on each one.

It will be five years this year that my Mum passed away and even last month on Mother's Day, just looking through photos of my Mum, I felt cheated she was taken too soon. I cried and felt all the initial grief reappear. I wanted to see my Mum and bring her flowers and chocolates, and my heart felt broken that I couldn't and never will.

People say, "Time is a healer." I think we have no choice but to get on with life; it's just very different now and always will be yet knowing that one day we will be reunited. I find comfort in knowing my Mum was very proud of us and is willing us on from above.

I'm also extremely lucky to have amazing friends and family who have been by my side and are still there for the sad days. I also see many signs Mum is around: feathers, butterflies, and songs suddenly come on the radio; all are a comfort, and I also know Mum is no longer in pain or discomfort and can rest in peace.

CHAPTER EIGHTEEN

CRYING

I didn't realise until grieving that crying came in many different forms, each with what seems to have its agenda attached to it. I experienced various types of crying, but all had the same agenda: a much-needed release to be able to recover.

There is the silent cry, where you sit with the stillness of tears rolling down your face with an overwhelming sense of sadness and the fear of dealing with stuff to the loud, wailing, ugly, snotty-faced cry. One thing for sure is that another emotion will take place when the cry is over. After this release, even if it has worn you out so you feel ready to rest, or a release which you can pick yourself up knowing it had to come out, it had been there waiting to burst through, literally like a floodgate. Or you may be in a numb stage where the tears aren't falling. Don't worry, they will, and we must let them.

We are all different, so crying doesn't have a timetable, even though we sometimes feel we must stop ourselves.

We feel the sting, blink the tears back, and reverse the process because we are uncomfortable letting it out. This is okay; we all do it, as long as it's not a constant thing we do to ourselves, as it has to come out at some point.

Sometimes, we cannot cry and find ourselves waiting patiently for it to happen. It is something that will happen to all of us, and this can happen in the numb stage of grieving. It must happen, and it will. The opposite of that is when you cry so much you feel you could fill a river, and you are actually scared you will never stop.

We need to cry to heal, so it should never be apologised for. It should never be mocked. Just a gentle nod of acknowledgement is sometimes all it takes if you see someone crying. It shouldn't leave anyone feeling uncomfortable. Know when to let things be for yourself and others. Realise we are all different on this, and some may want comfort when they are crying or just to be left alone, so communicate and let people know.

I remember being in a situation after losing my mother where a friend came to see me a few days later. She got really upset as I was a young Mum with three children, and she was saying, "This shouldn't be happening to you."

I know she was looking at me as if to say, 'Why are you not upset, not crying?' I was devastated, of course, but crying has a whole life of its own. When we are grieving, we realise this and that it's okay as long as, at some point, the tears are the same as the emotion that we must deal with. The tears will come.

I remember another time I was going to a support group for people who had specifically lost someone by taking their own life. Before I entered the room I was crying, as I walked in the room to see so many others in the same position as myself was overwhelming. I felt like I cried like I never had before. Being with people who totally understood my pain felt so powerful. The release was immense, and after I left the group, I felt a strange combination of exhaustion and being lighter simultaneously. Something had shifted, and it was all part of my healing journey.

So, cry, cry, and cry some more. It's natural, and it's okay. We do it for a reason. Give yourself permission to let it out. It's worth it.

Karen's story

Grieving is like a rollercoaster. One day, you are crumbling, and the next day, you're okay.

For me, when I was grieving the loss of my mum, I wanted the whole world to stop because I felt like I had stopped, and I couldn't understand. I felt frustrated even when I could hear people chatting and laughing while walking by my house. I felt like a piece of me was missing.

Grief rips through you and leaves you feeling stripped raw. The hole softens in time, but it always remains, for where there is deep grief, there is great love. You should never be ashamed of grief, judge it, or rush it. It is better to acknowledge, listen, feel, and sit with the pain; life must go on. Remember the love; this is where the healing will begin.

Always reach out to your nearest and dearest when you feel grief is too difficult to handle. They may not be able to take away the pain, but it helps to talk through your sadness and think about the happy memories shared. Over the years, when you lose so many family members, you feel the hole becoming bigger with so much sadness, but through each loss, you feel you get a bit stronger as a person. The tears still flow, but you think more of the happy memories you have shared and hold them close to your heart.

Everybody's grief is different, as we are all different. We all find a way of coping in our own way.

I AM READY TO LET GO OF...

CHAPTER NINETEEN

DRIVING LESSONS OF GRIEF

The brain takes us to such hard places in grief. I realised over time that I could think the same thoughts as before, and I didn't always have to attach them to grief. Instead, I was in control of my thoughts, working through their wildness, not letting them be attached to every thought I had or allowing grief joyriding on my every thought. It didn't have to feel so extreme all the time with it allowing it to control every situation I was in. Or all parts of my life, even parts that the loved one I had lost that was sometimes never involved in or they were never with me on certain occasions socially or at work. The person I loved may have gone, but my mind and all those things that happened when they were here were still the same. I guess it's part of moving on and accepting the grieving process.

Here is an example that may help. I was having a meal out with some friends not long after I lost my son-in-law. In my head, I spent the whole evening missing and yearning for him to still be with us, my thoughts kidnapped. I was not present but trying to act as if I were. I did not have the freedom to go with the flow of the conversation and enjoy my time with my friends. It wasn't until I got home and began to consider this that I recognised I had spent a whole night missing him when I was in a situation where he would never have been there anyway. I then worked through this and thought the next time I did something with my friends again, I would permit myself to have a break from grieving to be present.

Of course, it takes time, but by being gentle with ourselves and working through grief, these times will come. It is a constant reminder that we must give ourselves space and deal with it to achieve our desired outcome. We jump back and forth in our minds, trying to achieve how we want to feel, but we will get there. Imagine getting into a car without having any lessons and expecting to be able to drive and arrive safely at our destination. It would be impossible and be a wild ride fraught with danger and uncertainty. You must have lessons for the car to run smoothly by being in control and navigating your journey. Grieving is the same; we aren't experts in the beginning, and we can't run our lives the same straight way we were. We must go through the work and learn how to navigate our feelings. Then, our journey takes us along a smoother road. We'll keep hitting bumps, but we will get to our destination and a life of fulfilment again.

We have memories, so we hold on to them like precious gems. The day we realise that no one can take these away, we can gain comfort from them. Allowing ourselves to enjoy them takes time to get to this stage of grieving, and we can get snippets of it that give us hope. After working through the grief, it can feel comforting to feel a beautiful memory of a loved one we have lost. That memory is peaceful and a wonderful place to be. For a while we have arrived at a destination we want to be at.

Dale's story

I remember when my Nana died, all my family were panicking about how I would deal with losing her as I was very close to her, but I didn't feel as though it hit me as hard as I thought. I was out partying all the time as I was only twenty-five, so I think I masked my feelings.

The next big loss in my life was when I lost my Dad to cancer. I was expecting it as he was terminally ill. After he had passed away, I saw people older than he was walking on the streets, people I didn't know, and I felt angry he wasn't still here and felt really upset. I hadn't spent a lot of time with my Dad as he wasn't around when I was growing up. Still, we got closer as I became an adult - working and socialising together. He was my Dad, and I felt really sad.

Then I lost my Mum. I felt I had grieved for my Mum three times before she died as she was very poorly and in pain the last few years of her life. We were called to the hospital on numerous occasions to say she wouldn't make it through the night, so it was a rollercoaster. When the night came when she passed away, I actually felt as ready as she did for her to be out of pain and felt relieved when she finally passed away; of course, I was devastated, but relief was my first reaction. Afterwards, I was gutted that I would never see her again. It's upsetting again to think about it, even though it was seven years ago.

My next big loss was my son-in-law, a different sort of grief from any I had experienced. He had taken his own life, and I found him. I went through complete shock and devastation, and there had been no warning, nothing. I feel as though I have been through every emotion with this grief - anger, hurt, missing him, loving him, complete devastation in every way is how I describe it. But I must keep moving forward and spend as much time with my grandchildren doing all I can for them, and my family helps me in this process.

CHAPTER TWENTY

FEELINGS AROUND GRIEF

When we lose a person we love, it is a long process of working through our feelings and the stages to get through to the point of living again and being able to have beautiful memories as an enjoyable moment and not just be painful for us. Looking at it like this helps to understand how hard it is, how far you may have come, and perhaps be aware of some of the emotions you still must work through.

When we lose someone, we are thrown into the unknown cycle. I remember being told when we first lose a loved one that our body releases a natural anesthetic. It's the body's way of allowing you to cope with the intense feelings in the first few days. It is when this starts to wear off our feelings come through taking us into the unknown and expecting our wounded self to unravel itself to be again the person we were. That may be trying to laugh again, feel alive, or just feel okay. We know the reality is we won't be the same person after dealing with grief. Day-to-day life changes until we can travel alongside grief and work through it in a way to feel ourselves again.

There is no right or wrong way to unravel these emotions - just aim to work through them healthily while being kind to yourself. Forty-eight hours after my Mum passed away, I remember feeling really strong, yet it was all so painful. I couldn't believe, through all my pain, that I was still here, breathing and living, as it felt as if this pain wasn't survivable. This feeling of strength didn't last, but I knew it was inside me, and so I had the potential to feel it again. I think things like this take a while to realise when we reflect on what we have dealt with and still be here to tell our grieving journey to help others who are feeling as we are.

We must feel the emotions that come and go with grieving to work through them, not holding onto them and letting them go to get to a safe place and feel an inner peace we are worthy of. Once we have worked through them, they may try and stay with us in a way that brings us down; we can slowly start to dismiss those thoughts, safely knowing we have worked through them, replacing them with a positive one away from grieving. We are worthy of being happy and coming out the other side of these emotions; we deserve this and to let go of the guilt we experience after losing someone. This takes time, and we cannot rush the process, but we keep rolling with the waves that grief keeps hitting us with while working through the emotions and letting them go so we feel healed, lighter and happier.

Being around people with whom you can be yourself is very healing. People who let your feelings be and let you grieve when you want to provide a perfect grieving place. Feeling the love and comfort of a bubble of people who know you, get you, and understand you without judgment is a blessing.

The grieving process to recovery is like the worst homework in the world, as you have no choice but to live alongside the grieving. When I was on my counselling course, in one of my journals, I wrote of a technique I used while grieving, and my tutor said it was a helpful and healing way to deal with emotions. Sometimes, we are not in a place to be able to fully grieve at that moment, such as being back at work in a meeting or being around people we don't feel comfortable enough to let it all out with, and then we are flooded with emotions. I used to put them in an imaginary box in my brain, knowing I would have to open the box when it felt right to work through those emotions. To move forward, it was a coping technique that worked for me. It allowed me to deal with the world, and when I was in a comfortable place, I could grieve with myself or the people I wanted to grieve with.

This only came with a bit of practice to control it and wasn't something I could do in the early stages of grieving, but it helped me immensely to be checking in on myself and to make sure at some point I worked through whatever thought, feeling, emotion or trigger I had put in my imaginary box, in turn helping me heal and feel not so heavy with grief. Emotions to work through can seem impossible to fast-track and sometimes feel like they are never-ending. A whole new set of emotions then surprises us with the realising truth that it's an ongoing process.

The shock

The loss

The anxiety

The dreams

The intrusive thoughts

The initial relief

The images we see

The regret

The denial

The fear

The pain

The depression

The hurt

The loneliness

The disruptive sleep

The numbness

The crying

The anger

The loneliness

The missing

The physical pain

The guilt

The isolation

Seeing some of the emotions listed like this is a realisation of all we go through when grieving. The way these come and go through the different stages of grieving, sometimes crowding our minds to a point of us fighting through trying to make sense of it all.

As we try so hard to keep our heads above water, it can be easy to forget to talk, communicate, check in on each other, remember positive memories, and work through feelings together. We must grieve alone but supporting one another through the process can give us so much strength. It can help us not feel so alone and feel a real closeness when talking about the person we have lost. Of course, it takes time and effort sometimes to get together to talk, not always knowing what emotions might come up. Some might take us by surprise and might not align with what others are saying, but it's good to work through them together.

It helps us realise there is no right or wrong and comforts us that we are all grieving. Respecting what someone else is feeling and the strength we can gain is really helpful, giving us a new layer of love for each other in all we are going through together.

It helps to sometimes sit with these feelings, to feel them; if we don't work through them, we can experience delayed grief. This can be beneficial to a point if you are dealing with practical matters, but it's important to give yourself the space and time to feel them and grieve your loss to be able to heal and move forward.

Jacob's story

The first loss I remember was my Grandad, my Dad's father. I was a young boy and remember seeing my Dad crying his eyes out in bed. I didn't really understand it; it upset me seeing my Dad cry and brought me to tears.

My next loss was my Nana, my Dad's Mum. I expected it as she was often ill and was always in and out of the hospital, so when she actually passed away, I was really upset, but I had prepared myself.

Then I lost my brother-in-law. I came home from work after a normal day, and my Mum was worried; she said Chloe and Dad had gone to see where he was working because he hadn't answered his phone. I thought he would be fine, so I took a shower. When I came out, everything changed. I heard my Mum scream Chloe's name. I panicked, and my Mum told me he had taken his own life. I walked off, pacing around; knowing his sons were in the other room. I felt like I had a panic attack as I had never experienced a feeling like this before.

I walked into the other room, and his older son was smiling, asking why I was running around (he didn't know anything at this point). I knew I had to stay calm for him. My other sister came over after my Mum called her, and she took the boys home. I kept pacing around, telling myself it wasn't true.

A while later, Chloe, family, and friends were all at the house. It was like reliving it repeatedly when someone else came through the door. Talking about it now still upsets me, so I would rather not talk about it. Sometimes, I cope with it by not thinking about it. I know I block some of it out, but hopefully, in time, I can find it easier.

WHAT COMFORTS ME IN MY GRIEF?

CHAPTER TWENTY-ONE

RESPECT EACH OTHER'S GRIEF

Our relationship with the person we have lost is unique, and it is never the same as the relationship with the next person. As these relationships are all different, different feelings can come up at various times and in other periods in our lives, and we have different grieving patterns. There is a grieving format one is supposed to follow - the natural cycle of grief and pain.

People talk of the five stages of grief:

Denial

Anger

Bargaining

Depression

Acceptance

But grief is unpredictable; it's a wave of emotions that can hit us at any given time like a punch in the face. It comes out of nowhere, ready to take us down again and again. It takes us by surprise when we least expect it, wherever we go, and follows us like a stalker we can't get rid of. Sometimes, we can hold it back, push it back into the grief box in our brain it popped out of. This is okay temporarily, but we must deal with these emotions. Pushing them back in the box and not working through grief means it will spill out harder, unhealthier, and more painful in the future.

Working through grief takes time and hard work. It is like making a long journey without a sat nav, working through a network of feelings, some you never knew you had, trying to make sense of it all to get your life back on track. You aim to feel a set of positive emotions and find a way to navigate the negative thoughts that are weighing and dragging you down.

You are you, and I am I. No one knows us better than ourselves. We must be kind to ourselves, respect each other's grief, and help ourselves work through what we need to do.

We may not know instantly; our grief will feel different on different days. Some feelings may be familiar, and some may be new. This may change what we think. We may get stuck in a part of the grieving process and cannot move forward. We may realise at this point that we need help.

Just keep checking in on yourself and know when you need to speak up and reach out. This is always okay, not a weakness, but a strength. Knowing you have recognised this within yourself and are doing something about it is highly commendable.

Remember, the sun rises every morning. Each new day is a day to do something different, feel different, and think differently. If the day before didn't work for you, keep going one step at a time. We can do this. Learn from your own thoughts what works for you.

Sharon's story

I lost my Mum in August 2020 during Lockdown; she was ninety-two. She lived to a good age and had a good life. This is what I would say to people when I told them that she had passed away before they had chance to say it, because they did say it to me, many times. Being ninety-two does not make it any easier; it means that you have had them in your life for longer. It means that they have been there for you for longer, you have loved them for longer, and now that adult who had always been there for you has gone. I didn't care that she was a good age or that she had had a good life; she was my Mum, and I wasn't ready to lose her, even at fifty-two. My Dad passed away when I was two years old, so it had been the two of us for fifty years, and for the last seventeen years of that, she had my daughter, too. We were her world.

I did everything I could to keep her safe during COVID-19. I remember receiving a text from a work colleague saying that the first case was reported in our town on 7th March 2020. We were on our weekly shopping trip to Morrisons. That was the last time she went to a shop of any kind. I visited her every other day, and she stayed in her armchair while I did bits for her, went shopping, collected prescriptions, fed the birds and hedgehogs, and wiped down with anti-bac all the surfaces that I had touched. I did everything I could to keep her safe. 'Stay in the chair,' I would say so that I could keep my distance. I still feel guilty about this almost four years later. Why? Because I blame myself for not noticing how she was deteriorating over the months that followed. I couldn't tell she was struggling to get her breath when she walked up the stairs or ate less; I was just concerned about two-metre distancing to keep her safe.

A doctor admitted her to the hospital on the 27th of July, and I still didn't realise how serious it was. I had just got engaged, and I was getting married in October; not for one second did I think that she wouldn't be there. I left her at the hospital, told her I loved her, and I would see her soon. That was the last time I saw her. I was able to FaceTime with her a couple of times, and it was so hard; I could see her getting frailer and frailer, and there was nothing I could do. I couldn't visit and could tell the video calls upset her. I showed her a video of me trying on my wedding dress, but deep down, I knew she wouldn't see me in the dress again.

The call came just before four a.m. I thanked the nurse for letting me know. I was very businesslike about it all; I just felt numb. I carried on as normal. I'm strong; that's what I do. I'm there for everyone. I don't talk about my feelings; I support others with theirs.

Then it started.

'She had a good life. She was a good age.'

'No', I wanted to scream at them, 'she was my Mum. I don't care how old she was; it makes no difference. I am heartbroken', but I just smiled and nodded. People would tell me they knew how I felt and knew what I was going through. No - they knew how they felt about their experiences; they knew what they went through, and whilst I was sympathetic that they had suffered loss, they did not know how I was feeling. It wasn't long before the anger came. I needed answers, and I couldn't get any. I felt and still do feel guilty for not noticing how she was becoming frailer. It still makes me sad that she has missed so much that she would have been so proud of - the wedding, my daughter's A levels, university, my stepdaughter's career, their eighteenth and twenty-first birthdays; she would have been so proud of them both.

I was still smiling and nodding to the good life, good age comments when, a week after my Mum passed away, my Father-in-law was diagnosed with cancer; he passed away in December 2020.

We then lost my Mother-in-law to cancer in March 2021. I didn't have a chance to grieve, and it took me over twelve months to realise this; I was supporting my husband and sister-in-law through such a difficult time. They were both a lot younger than me, and their parents were only in their late sixties and early seventies. It was different from my Mum's because she was older. It was different but wasn't as she was still my Mum. I found myself dismissing any conversations regarding my grief and focusing on the feelings of my family, who needed my support.

I can't remember how I came to contact the bereavement counsellor. I needed to get the feelings out that were spinning around in my head; someone described it as a washing machine, which is a great description. I have used CBT strategies in the past, but there was just too much to break down and work through. I find lists and writing things down really useful, but I couldn't write this down. I experienced feelings and thoughts that I had never had before, anger and horrible thoughts about friends and family that I could never say out loud. I felt so much guilt about the anger about not being in control and not being able to take control, the other feelings and the absolutely awful thoughts that I was having about the people that I love.

The counsellor also described it well, and such a simple analogy really helped me. She said it was like shaking a lemonade bottle. Eventually, the bubbles will build up, and if they keep building without loosening the lid, the bottle will explode. So gradually, I would tell her about the horrible thoughts, the anger, the guilt, and it was like gently opening that bottle lid a little bit at a time to release the pressure. She helped me to realise that all my feelings were okay. You can't help how you feel and the thoughts that spin around in your head.

The really bad thoughts that I had were okay. I was grieving, and the thoughts and feelings were all part of that.

I miss her and think about her every day. No matter how old you are, sometimes you just need a grown-up to hug you and tell you everything will be okay, or you're doing a good job, or simply just for that hug that no one else can give you. I still miss that. With my daughter's graduation in a few months, this will be another event to overcome, happiness but tinged with some sadness.

A few weeks ago, I realised something when I was trying to help someone that I care about with the grieving pain they were going through. The pain does ease very gradually, but I don't think you realise that because you forget how painful and all-consuming it was in the beginning.

SOMETHING I AM LEARNING TO ACCEPT IS...

CHAPTER TWENTY-TWO

MY GRIEVING LIFE

Be kind to yourself.

From the age of fourteen, my first experience of grief, I have lost many family members. I feel as though grief wrapped around my whole life.

There have been periods in between to process my grief to then find myself on another journey of losing someone again. The thing I have learnt during all of this, after times of being thrown into this road of grieving you never want to be on, is realising that the grief life is full of highs and lows.

I have learnt that when you are grieving, to try and still do the things you enjoy and make your life fulfilling. It is very important to continue to do so, to keep yourself feeling like you. Of course, this is hard when every fibre of our being hurts, and we feel like shutting down, but we must realise we must carry on. Also, we should do these things without guilt, knowing our loved ones would want us to continue. Doing things we enjoyed before feels different when we are grieving. If we allow the negative guilt voices we hear telling us to stop or 'I shouldn't enjoy myself', they can be really damaging. Of course, in the early stages of grieving, it feels impossible and the physical pain we feel, and the exhaustion needs working through first. However, we must still permit ourselves to be as we were before, which is okay, and if we keep pushing forward, we'll come out the other side of grieving.

It can feel easier sometimes to say no and keep ourselves shut away, but doing positive things like meeting with friends and doing enjoyable things for ourselves, going out for a nice meal, climbing mountains, going to the cinema, or whatever that may be, can be very beneficial in our healing. Keeping to our routine when we can and doing our familiar things makes us feel like us.

Loved ones would still only want the best for us. We must be in control of our self-care to be gentle with ourselves and remember who we were before our loss. We know we will never be the same, but we know how important it is not to lose our old selves.

Grief changes you, but we are in control of ourselves, and we must remember to control our thoughts and not let them control us. It's sometimes easier said than done, but replacing a negative thought straight away with a positive can help break this cycle; I remember the guilt

I have felt from laughing after loss and being hard on myself for having an emotion that's not attached to grief. I thought it was weird if I had a moment of enjoyment. We need to grieve but not be hard on ourselves, knowing every second is precious in our lives.

When those lights of hope come through, embrace them, as with the twists and turns of grief, it will change again. You are not forcing anything but tuning into a natural feeling of hope or happiness as it pops up, making you feel lighter and gaining a moment of peace. It is invaluable. Grief is hard enough without us being harder on ourselves; make it normal to be kind to ourselves.

WRITE A LETTER TO YOUR LOVED ONE

CHAPTER TWENTY-THREE

EMOTIONS

We must work through emotions, whether we love or hate them. Like a subject at school that must be studied to get the result we want, we must work hard to get our qualifications in life. We must feel our emotions and deal with them to understand and cope with them.

Moving forward from them is more challenging than graduating. Once we have learned to master a topic, it's ongoing, like a lifetime of lessons in emotions. Of course, sometimes, we don't have time to study our well-being and emotions. We dismiss them, stopping ourselves from feeling them. We feel numb, quickly replacing them with another feeling. But like doing an exam without revision, the results will not be good. We must work through them to feel what they are telling us, revise them often, and use our thought processes to think our way out of them.

Some of these feelings are so strong that we feel trapped in them, not knowing where the door is to release them or work through them. A certain emotion or feeling we can't work through may need help, just like any other form of work we struggle with - our minds and mental health are no different. This helps us and gives us the skills to work it out and keep moving forward. That may be talking to a friend, getting professional help, or spending time on us to get to know our new selves and how they make us feel.

If we constantly ignore working through these emotions and stages of grief, they will come back to bite us. They will come out in other ways that can be unhealthy and harder to deal with. It's a ride we are on and can't get off. So, when an emotion appears, we know it is kinder to us to deal with it. In the end, we will have a less rocky journey and eventually gain more peace within ourselves, achieving the result in life we deserve.

HOW HAVE MY EMOTIONS CHANGED?

AFTER

WHEN SOME TIME HAS PASSED

CHAPTER TWENTY-FOUR

CONTINUING FORWARD

We have now been on the grieving journey for some time; we have got to know and recognise what our grieving feels like and work through it; we have got to know our triggers, the way they make us act, and how to work with them and through them.

Next, we must focus on what we have now in our lives and try to place our attention on the good memories of the past. This takes time and effort to get to this point. It doesn't happen overnight; the snippets of it as we work through our grief, the feelings of hope instead of despair, make us realise it's possible, leading us in the right direction. With the unpredictability of grief, it can still creep up behind us and give us a bad day. This is normal, but when we have worked through those emotions, we can get through it, knowing it will pass, allowing us to keep moving forward.

Being stuck in one of the cycles of grief may require us to get help. It's normal to keep dipping in and out. Still, we must keep moving with these emotions, not feeling glued to grief, and pull ourselves away from the heavy burden of it through all our hard work to feel free from constant, deep pain.

Remember how far you have come; we are living proof we can come through grief. It will change us, challenge, and keep trying to put us down. No one ever said it was easy, but we can do it by keeping moving forward with all we have learnt and knowing we deserve to be here living how we want to.

CHAPTER TWENTY-FIVE

LIVE YOUR LIFE

We must work through our grief to come out the other side, but I have learnt that we can still live a life while doing so. Grieving will be there to rear its ugly head when you least expect it, coming in waves. When these waves are calm, it's a time to reflect on our lives and look at what we have and are truly grateful for. Losing someone magnifies this, and we must keep hold of these thoughts, as these positives will help us cope and feel stronger. These don't have to be massive things in our lives. Often, the smaller things will humble us and give us a feeling of peace.

Many have come out the other side of grieving with a new zest for life, realising there are no guarantees. So, if able, they have given themselves permission to do what they haven't thought possible before. They've seen things and circumstances through different eyes, providing them with a different perspective and helping them reach decisions they had struggled with previously to give them the best outcomes of their own lives.

Remember, we are here to live a fulfilled, happy, peaceful life ourselves. This is in no way selfish, and we shouldn't feel guilty as a result. We need to give ourselves permission and be kind to ourselves to live our lives and try to keep doing this alongside our grief.

If we don't live our lives to our fullest potential and do what makes us happy, there will not be any more beautiful memories created for the future and for ourselves and others to look back on. It's okay to live your life while grieving.

CHAPTER TWENTY-SIX

POSITIVE AFFIRMATIONS

Affirmations are positive-loaded phrases or statements used to challenge negative, unhelpful thoughts, which we often experience when we are grieving.

We can use these to change our thought processes, help us through hard times, increase our positive thoughts, manifest goodness, make positive life changes and boost our self-esteem.

Write an affirmation and repeat it to yourself several times in the morning to help your thought process start positively.

Keep it positive, short and personal.

For example:

> **I am stronger than I think.**
>
> **I have all I need to cope inside of me.**
>
> **I will take care of my mind.**

Try it and see if it works for you.

WRITE A POSITIVE AFFIRMATION TO YOURSELF FOR WHEN YOU'RE OVERWHELMED BY GRIEF

CHAPTER TWENTY-SEVEN

THE IMPORTANCE OF SELF-CARE

Self-care doesn't have to be extravagant. The smallest things can rejuvenate us, leaving us feeling clearer and able to carry on.

What is self-care? It is the practice of protecting our happiness and well-being, particularly when we are under stress - looking after ourselves physically, mentally and spiritually.

We may do this really well before being thrown into grieving. Still, sometimes, the grieving process can lead to a feeling that we don't deserve it or that it's unimportant to fit into our grieving life. This is untrue. It is a must that we look after our physical and mental well-being to get us through the grieving process.

I realised the importance of self-care after having a particularly bad couple of weeks of grieving. Firstly, I noticed it made me overthink those around me, how they were feeling, and the importance of checking in on your loved ones. I asked if they were doing okay because, from the outside, no one knew I was having a bad time. While you permit others, looking after your well-being without guilt is okay. It also made me realise the harsh reality of being responsible for our well-being. Whether that's arranging to meet friends, so we aren't so isolated. Or to have a massage, get our hair done, go for a walk, read a book, go on holiday, or reach out for other help we may need, like counselling or a support group. The importance of asking others how they are may mean we can navigate through these hard times, helping each other, talking and communicating to work through it, giving ourselves permission and others the importance of self-care to remove any guilt from it completely. It is a part of grieving that should be given a big priority.

One thing we can do is be there for ourselves. Read that again - to be there for ourselves. Think of all the kind words you would say to a friend or family member grieving or struggling. What would we say? We are important enough to say these words to ourselves, to be kind and care for ourselves, to treat ourselves as we would the ones we love, and to love ourselves enough to heal and live the life we know we can.

I realised I could also distract myself by practising self-care, changing my mindset, playing music, writing, and remembering what I enjoy. I should not lose myself in the grieving process. Doing things for yourself will help keep you feeling like you and grab hold of good moments.

We must reach a place where we focus on the good memories of our lost ones and are grateful for what we have in the here and now. We must move forward with a positive mindset to live a life filled with our hearts full of love for ourselves, the way the ones we lost would want us to feel. To do this, we must take care of ourselves.

Taking time for ourselves empowers us to decide about our health and well-being. Self-care is literally caring about ourselves. When you really think about it - without caring about ourselves and our well-being, it is impossible to care for someone else. We often do things for others but do not give ourselves the care and support we need. It's much more recognised now that this is what we need to do to live and deal with life itself - even gentle reminders to eat and sleep well to function. We must ask ourselves why this sometimes feels like we shouldn't and find it hard, why we feel guilty for giving ourselves the time.

The key to this is managing your time appropriately and getting the balance right. Therefore, give yourself permission to know that your self-care is also a priority. It may be simply allowing ourselves time to sit and have that cup of tea; it can be as simple as allowing yourself to watch TV for an hour. You must fit it in to be your number-one fan! It will make the struggles of life and grieving more manageable.

It seems so easy to see from the outside what we feel others may need without looking at our own needs. We are good at telling others to look after themselves; we must say it to ourselves, too. We tell others to take time to do something they enjoy, such as they must continue to take part in a hobby, but not do it ourselves. We need to treat ourselves as we would others. Normalising this with ourselves will help us to achieve real inner peace.

In addition to the self-care we give ourselves, we must recognise when we may need professional help. We must care about ourselves. It's only as I have gotten older and lost loved ones that I have realised how much self-care and taking time out for ourselves can help in our grieving process. The first time we find ourselves alone, with the silence and not with people, can be hard. We are left with our own thoughts, but not only does this give us time to process them, but if we enable ourselves to do it within self-care quality time, it can be very healing and beneficial.

I was introduced to yoga Nidra while in the early stages of grieving my son-in-law. It's yoga for the mind - a form of meditation. A friend offered me a free session. It is a practice done by laying totally still and just listening. I couldn't believe its effect on my mind and body, easing me into the relaxation I had craved since losing him. It helped me to release tension, which melted away as I listened to the yoga teacher's calm, soothing voice instructing me through the practice. I will be forever grateful to my friend for introducing me to yoga Nidra. I continue to do this at home. You can find many sessions on YouTube or a private one-to-one session with someone qualified to guide you. Whatever your go-to is, a walk, a run, a massage, or a bubble bath, this time is healing, and you become aware of yourself and your thoughts. Feeling calmer can really help you move forward.

If self-care is new to you, here are a few ideas to help you be kind to yourself and use this as part of your healing process:

Walk

Yoga Nidra/meditation

Relax with a bubble bath

Have a healthy eating and sleep routine

Phone call with a friend

Read

Hobbies

Write

Get a massage/facial

Sit and focus on positivity and manifest

Manicure/pedicure

Have your hair done

Cook alone or with friends

Bake

Rest

Exercise

Join a support group

Get professional counselling

The list really is endless. The point is that it is something that you enjoy, that makes you feel good, and that relaxes you.

Always look after your emotional, physical, psychological, and spiritual health. This is a must while grieving and throughout life to achieve a sense of well-being.

SELF-CARE, WHAT AM I DOING FOR MYSELF?

CHAPTER TWENTY-EIGHT

DO YOU

Sometimes, it can feel like a contradiction, as we are being told by all kinds of people to 'be strong, you can do this, you've got this.'

This is unhealthy; just do you. As other's words can lead to comparing ourselves to others and how they are coping, feeling we should be the same way.

'Just because someone doesn't need medication or counselling - why should I?'

The simple answer is that we are all different, so what one is doing, another is not, can't, or doesn't find helpful. It's okay.

When you're grappling with grief, it's important to understand that it's not just okay, but it's completely normal to reach out for support. Whether that's a heart-to-heart with a friend or a professional consultation, you are the best judge of what you need. Recognising your needs and taking steps to meet them is a significant act of self-care and self-empowerment.

Gain comfort in the knowledge that before you and after you, others have done this, even if you don't know how. Thousands have had counselling, thousands need help, thousands have joined support groups, and thousands have been prescribed medication to help them; you are not alone.

One step can lead you on a journey, and then you will feel cushioned against your grieving. You deserve it to yourself to travel this grieving journey the way you need to and live the life you deserve. No one knows you better than yourself. You have all the answers somewhere to do you and what you need to do. Always believe in recognising this and in yourself.

NOW YOU'RE NOT HERE, MY BIGGEST MOTIVATION IS

CHAPTER TWENTY-NINE

SIGNS

Signs we believe are sent from a loved one after they have passed away can bring us comfort like no other when they aren't around. I have a friend who works within a funeral home and has over twenty years of experience within the industry. She has heard countless stories of things that have happened to people over the years after losing loved ones, each personal and relevant to each loss, demonstrated through a sign from their loved ones. It could be a feeling, situation, smell, seeing something, whatever it may be; I believe they are signs.

We don't have to understand how or why; we must accept it for what it is. Whether you believe in a sign or not, it's important to respect what another person says to you if they believe they have had one.

Over the years, I've had many personal signs, usually soon after a loved one has passed. I would like to share a few with you.

My son-in-law occasionally enjoyed a game of roulette at the casino after a night out; he and my daughter would all enjoy the fun with their friends. After he passed away, his wife, my other daughter and my sister were at their house watching TV. Around midnight, a late-night casino programme came on the TV. It was a roulette game. As they looked at the spinning wheel on the screen, the first number the ball landed in was the first. When my son-in-law played roulette, he used his first son's birthday, his first lucky number. They all commented and looked in disbelief. As the second spin happened, the ball landed on his next lucky number, his second son's birthday; 'wow, what a coincidence', they all said. With the next three spins of the wheel, the balls landed on his next three lucky favourite numbers he always played! All his lucky numbers, a total of five, were played in the correct order. This was a sign to us that he was okay.

When my auntie was poorly and in the last stages of her life, she was living with my cousins, where she was being loved and cared for until she passed. She was an amazing lady, and there was an interesting conversation about her in her last few weeks. There was a decorative metal wall art flower hung up behind the TV. It was almost said in jest, as she had a fantastic sense of humour, that she would knock that off the wall after she had passed to let them know she was okay; a few weeks after her passing, it did indeed fall off the wall and slip down the back of the TV. We saw this as a sure sign she was indeed okay.

There are many signs, some really small, such as the floating of a white feather in front of us or a feeling we can't explain and mostly we aren't expecting; we just have a sense we know it is a definite sign. When it happens, it feels good. It doesn't always happen and again this is okay, it is something we can't question or control. When it does, it brings a level of comfort that is hard to describe, so don't question it. Embrace it.

MY FAVOURITE MEMORIES ARE...

CHAPTER THIRTY

THE HERE AND NOW

If we do not focus on today, we can spend so much time worrying about the future because of what has happened in the past. This snatches away our lives. We must be present to enjoy today and not let our grieving process completely take over our whole being.

This is how it feels initially, and we must work through all our emotions to be present. Of course, the big wave of grief will keep appearing, but we must remind ourselves we are here, and that life goes by quickly. We must live it to our fullest and love ourselves as the ones we have lost would want us to. It is sometimes a lot harder to do this than we think. We must constantly learn and train ourselves not to get carried away by worrying and overthinking. It's not easy to do this, and it takes practice and constant reminders from us that it is an easier way to live.

It made me feel like I had to be present and only live for today, as nothing is guaranteed. However, I am making continuous progress in not worrying about the past and not trying to predict the future. I know it's a happier and more positive place to live today. What is happening now at this moment? We can collect our thoughts, ground ourselves, sit, and go through our minds, finding all we love and are grateful for to help us stay focused and positive.

Try this: Fast-forward yourself to the future, say twenty years from now. Now, look back. Have those years been how you wanted to live them? Have you appreciated your own life and been present, enjoying each moment you can as you should?

If not, you would be so angry with yourself for not being present and for stressing what may or may not happen. You must free yourself of this to be present and at peace and to give yourself the life you deserve.

WHAT AM I GRATEFUL FOR?

CHAPTER THIRTY-ONE

GETTING TO KNOW THE NEW YOU

Losing someone you love changes you; it must be the most stressful thing in life to deal with. Knowing your grieving self and getting to know the new you are beneficial to coping day-to-day. We can miss our old selves and lives immensely, which is why we are getting to grips with how we will function and live without the person we have lost.

It allows you to understand that having a bad day is totally normal. I know myself and how I grieve that although a bad day takes me by total surprise, sometimes it is normal, and I hope to feel different again the next day. It's normal to have these days for years to come, but we manage them through the coping mechanisms we have taught ourselves and with the confidence that they will pass.

Of course, if these days become unbearable and are consecutive and you feel unable to manage them, reaching out for help may be needed, and that's okay.

Sometimes, that reach can be phoning a friend or getting professional help; it's your journey.

Be gentle with yourself and keep assessing yourself along your journey, learning what is needed. Never be afraid to ask for help. There is no right or wrong. Being stuck in a negative part of this grieving cycle can feel very lonely, but you can always work through pain. To see a glimmer of light reminds you a dark day will lift. Never forget this: this feeling will pass. It will come and go, so push through. You will come out the other side, turning a corner on your grief again, walking alongside it, dealing with it, smashing through those emotions, feeling a sense of relief again and another step closer to feeling more at peace with your mind.

Gradually, as you are living in your new world of grief, using the inner strength you never knew you had, take a lesson from this. Let it empower you, knowing that in your hardest times, it will change again, and your feelings will become manageable again. Let these be moments you can reflect on when you need to know you will get through even the toughest times, reminding yourself how far you have already come.

MOMENTS OF LIGHT AND HOPE THAT HAVE HELPED ME

CHAPTER THIRTY-TWO

COMING THROUGH THE OTHER SIDE OF GRIEF

As survivors of grief, we are our own version of superheroes, as we will get there in the end. Travelling along on our paths of grief, falling off the curb along the way, and picking ourselves back up constantly can leave us feeling exhausted. We carry on as the waves of grief keep knocking us down until suddenly, one of the waves feels less harsh and more like a ripple of emotion, giving us hope we can do this. Then, it shocks us that we remember a fond memory of the person we lost. It causes us to smile a little and feel hope.

However, grieving gives you the other superpower of being able to host a party of emotions at once. Crying, laughing, and feeling anger can all be part of the norm in the grieving cycle, meaning you're not going crazy. Still, those emotional waves take a bit longer to process our thoughts, come through the other side, and not feel so overwhelmed with it all.

We may wonder if we have come out the other side of grieving. For some, it takes longer than others; for others, we don't come out the other side, but walking peacefully at the side of it is all okay. I think one of the true signs that shows you are healing is that you can celebrate the memories of your loved one in a way that feels happy and joyful while it's natural for you to want them to be there. The feeling that our memory isn't weighed down with pain and hurt is not a sudden process. Little rays of hope and light sprinkle through, and you know it feels different within yourself. It could be the acceptance of the loss. Sometimes acceptance can feel like a daunting word and something we can never achieve in a way we would like, but having a sense that you are doing okay, doing your best and all life isn't grief consumed is moving in the right direction, so don't worry about your grief timelines too much, as long as you are coping.

What's vital is living guilt-free, laughing again, and having genuine fun. It also means making new choices and feeling real purpose in your life again.

Realise that all we have are their precious memories. It takes a while to think of these with less pain, and while we are in the early stages of grieving when they appear and bring us happiness from the black cloud grief brings, it is so comforting. Everything we do in our lives becomes a memory; remember that. We must live recognising that yesterday is a memory; none of us can predict tomorrow, so we must try and enjoy each day, knowing that these two will become special moments we enjoy with our friends and family - the people we love. Let this thought help you be present and enjoy the here and now; often, thinking this is what the loved one we have lost would want can help. They hated seeing us sad when they were alive and wouldn't want us to be sad all the time now.

Look forward to the moments of happiness that come. There is no guilt to experience. It's our life, and we know how precious it is, so we must live it fully. Looking at the photos and memories on our phones brings us joy; we realise how lucky we are to have these pictures free to look at whenever we choose - beautiful memories in our hands at the click of a button. Years ago, it would be a case of waiting until we got home to get photo albums out and dusty boxes of photos to remind ourselves of wonderful times and memories.

Allow yourself to be loved and love others to feel free with your emotions.

For some, grief may never leave us. We must be able to do the above in our own lives. It has changed us. It is there, but we are not carrying it as a big load. We are running a life that feels happy alongside it. No one knows us better than we do. We all deserve to be happy. Grief puts the breaks on our lives, but we can and will come through it, learning and thriving once again in our new world.

THE AFTER ME

Grief is inside me.
Is this really happening?
Grief has got hold of me.
I need to let it go.
Grief has broken me.
I have to fix this.
Grief has taken my mind.
I need to unravel this.
Grief is still here.
It has shaped me.
Grief has changed me.
I will not fear the change.
I can now walk alongside my grief.

TO MY FAMILY AND FRIENDS

THANK YOU

I know I'm very lucky to be surrounded by amazing family and friends. I know this has helped me throughout my life in coping with my grief.

Many of whom have been kind enough to share their own stories of grief in this book.

I hope I have helped you all as much as you have helped me. You know who you all are. I want to thank you from the bottom of my heart, and as long as I'm here, I will continue to love and support you all as long as I can.

Love Marie x

HELPLINES AND SUPPORT

Samaritans
Helpline for whatever you are going through
Call 116 123 free 24 hours a day 365 days a year

SOBS
Survival of bereavement by suicide
Supporting anyone affected by suicide
0300 111 5065
WWW.uksobs.org

RoadPeace
Support after road death and injury
0800 160 1069
helpline@roadpeace.org

Winston's Wish
Help for children , teenagers and young adults (up to the age of 25) when their worlds turned upside down by grief
08088 020 021

Cruse
Bereavement support
0808 808 1677

LOROS
Support for terminally ill patients , families and carers in Leicestershire and Rutland
0116 231 3771
loros.co.uk

The Compassionate Friends
TCF a nationwide organisation for bereaved parents and sibling support after the death of a child
0345 123 2304
helpline@tcf.org.uk

NHS therapy and counselling services
Referral through GP or self-referral through NHS talking therapies online

All numbers and details correct of July 2024

CONNECT WITH ME

If you've felt inspired by this book,
please leave me a review on Amazon.

Please feel free to get in touch with me here via
my email: mariehbrown@btinternet.com